Trickster in Tweed

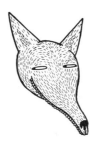

WRITING LIVES
Ethnographic Narratives

Series Editors:
Arthur P. Bochner & Carolyn Ellis
University of South Florida

Writing Lives: Ethnographic Narratives publishes narrative representations of qualitative research projects. The series editors seek manuscripts that blur the boundaries between humanities and social sciences. We encourage novel and evocative forms of expressing concrete lived experience, including autoethnographic, literary, poetic, artistic, visual, performative, critical, multi-voiced, conversational, and co-constructed representations. We are interested in ethnographic narratives that depict local stories; employ literary modes of scene setting, dialogue, character development, and unfolding action; and include the author's critical reflections on the research and writing process, such as research ethics, alternative modes of inquiry and representation, reflexivity, and evocative storytelling. Proposals and manuscripts should be directed to abochner@cas.usf.edu.

Volumes in this series:

Erotic Mentoring: Women's Transformations in the University
 Janice Hocker Rushing

Intimate Colonialism: Head, Heart, and Body in West African Development Work
 Laurie L. Charlés

Last Writes: A Daybook for a Dying Friend
 Laurel Richardson

Trickster in Tweed: My Quest for Quality in Faculty Life
 Thomas S. Frentz

Guyana Diaries: Women's Lives Across Difference
 Kimberly D. Nettles

Writing Qualitative Inquiry: Self, Stories, and Academic Life
 H. L. Goodall, Jr.

Trickster in Tweed

MY QUEST FOR QUALITY IN FACULTY LIFE

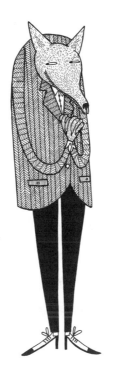

Thomas S. Frentz

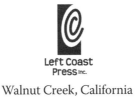

Left Coast
Press Inc.

Walnut Creek, California

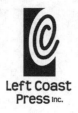

Left Coast Press Inc.

LEFT COAST PRESS, INC.
1630 North Main Street, #400
Walnut Creek, CA 94596
http://www.LCoastPress.com

ISBN   978-1-59874-317-3   Cloth
ISBN   978-1-59874-318-0   Paper

Library of Congress Cataloging-in-Publication Data
Frentz, Thomas S.
    Trickster in tweed : my quest for quality in faculty life / Thomas S. Frentz.
        p.   cm. — (Writing lives)
    Includes bibliographical references and index.
    ISBN 978-1-59874-317-3 (hardback : alk. paper)
    ISBN 978-1-59874-318-0 (pbk. : alk. paper)
1. Frentz, Thomas S.   2. College teachers—United States—Biography.   3. Organizational behavior—United States.   4. Cancer—Patients—Biography.   5. Self-realization—United States.   I. Title.
LA2317.F854A3 2008
378.1'2092—dc22
[B]   2008003541

Printed in the United States of America

⊖™ The paper used in this publication meets the minimum requirements of American National Standard for Information Sciences—Permanence of Paper for Printed Library Materials, ANSI/NISO Z39.48–1992.

08 09 10 11 12 5 4 3 2 1

Text Designer: Detta Penna
Copyeditor: Judith Johnstone
Indexer: Sally Brown

Contents

for Janice

Foreword

Writing Lives: Ethnographic Narratives publishes experimental forms of qualitative writing that blur boundaries between the social sciences and humanities. Books in this series feature concrete details of everyday life in which people are presented as complicated and vulnerable human beings who act and feel in complex, often unpredictable ways. As social agents constrained but not controlled by culture, the characters in these books tell stories that often show a dazzling human capacity to remake and reform cultural narratives.

We encourage authors in this series to write ethnography reflexively, weaving details about their own lives and relationships into the stories they tell about others. The series' authors seek to share interpretive authority by presenting layered accounts with multiple voices and by experimenting with unconventional forms of representation, including the fictional and the poetic. They try to stay open to surprise and to encourage challenges and revisions to their own interpretations. In these books, interpretive authority ultimately lies with the community of readers who engage the text. When these texts succeed, they encourage readers to feel, think about, and compare their own worlds of experience with those of the people they meet on the pages of these stories. In addition to stimulating a dialogue among academics across disciplinary lines, the accessible books in the *Writing Lives: Ethnographic Narratives* series can appeal to a wider public audience, especially people who can influence policy and implement social change.

In *Trickster in Tweed: My Quest for Quality in Faculty Life,* Tom Frentz wrestles with the alienation, demoralization, isolation, and anger he experienced over a lifetime as a university professor. Refusing to give up his quest for a meaningful, high quality life, or give in to the institutional depression that permeates American universities in the twenty-first century, Tom turns to personal narrative and autoethnography to better understand the emotional and institutional sources of his discontent and to fashion a new story for himself, one that would allow his own voice to flourish and make it possible for him to merge his heart with his head in both teaching and research.

To achieve these goals, Tom takes a sober and candid look at the past, revisiting painful moments of his childhood, adolescence, graduate education, progression though the academic ranks, professional disappointments, betrayals by colleagues and friends, a life-threatening cancer diagnosis, and the excruciating loss of the love of his life. His is not a heroic tale. Often—too often—he acts badly and suffers dire consequences, especially during the early years of his life as a professor. In many respects, his stories depict a torturous path toward self-understanding and self-transformation. As we read Tom's stories, we laughed, we cried and, occasionally, we shook our heads, not in disbelief but rather in a state of horrified recognition and familiarity.

Tom resists the temptation to blame everything on the culture of the university. He provides a trenchant critique of the "life of the mind," insisting that a high quality life cannot be lived only from the neck up, and revealing the troubling and self-defeating consequences of the competitive and cut-throat atmosphere of the university, which typically neglects the inner life of professors and discourages integration of the personal/emotional with the academic/intellectual. Tom's stories suggest that university culture is not fixed and unalterable. The culture depends largely, though not exclusively, on the choices individual professors make about what and how to teach, write, and build community and collegiality with each other. Too many of us react to the paralysis we feel, Tom argues, either with sheep-like dependence or wolf-like aggression. In either case, we take the easy way out. We let ourselves off the hook, blaming our misery exclusively on sources outside ourselves. Tom introduces a third animal-persona, the coyote/trickster, who sees an alternative to rebellion against, or submission to, authority. Accepting that he or she is both a part of and apart from debilitating authority structures, the trickster laces his actions and utterances with rule-bending humor and satire, destabilizing rigid organizational hierarchies and self-defeating conventions, collapsing oppositions, embracing paradoxes and contradictions, and showing the absurdity of unchallenged and unquestioned practices.

Professors are socialized to be critical. Ironically, however, few academics have focused a critical lens on their own lives as academics. We do not see ourselves as embedded in a strange subculture—the university—and only rarely do we talk with each other about this culture in profoundly self-critical ways. Though a few exceptions exist, most books on academic life have been written by retired professors after they left academic life, or have taken the form of humorous fictional satire meant to poke fun at academic culture.

Trickster in Tweed: My Quest for Quality in Faculty Life, breaks the mold. Written by a committed academic still teaching and publishing at the age of 69, and still trying to define the meaning and quality of his life, *Trickster* grapples with large and important issues at the heart of every academic life: our ethical responsibility to teach more than content to our students—to touch them emotionally, spiritually, and morally; the extraordinary difficulty of sustaining a passion for teaching and research over the entire course of an academic lifetime; the competitive practices and hierarchies that diminish trust and collegiality, encourage secrecy, gossip, and betrayal, and make nearly every faculty member feel like a fraud at times; the isolating cleavage between the personal and academic that discourages creativity and innovation; the ego-battering nature of an academic life; the corporate business model of efficiency that equates effective teaching with student ratings, and significant research with the sheer number of publications in peer-reviewed and sanctioned journals; and the idea that a faculty life is not a calling but a career in which each of us is obliged to market ourselves as an academic entrepreneur.

You will not like everything Tom Frentz says and does in the course of his academic life, though we expect you will admire his candor and courage. Regardless, you will at least have to ask yourself, where am I in this story? What can I do to make my academic life more meaningful, and of higher quality? How can I help my students and my colleagues achieve better lives? How can I contribute to making my university more humane, just, and fair? What ever happened to my dream of academic ecstasy?

Arthur P. Bochner and Carolyn S. Ellis
University of South Florida
Series Editors: Writing Lives

Preface

I began writing this story in January 2000, right after being diagnosed with cancer. Initially, I didn't think of what I was doing as autoethnographic scholarship, or any kind of scholarship for that matter. I was just scared and needed something to take my mind off my misery. So I figured writing a little something every day would not only be in keeping with both Anne Lamott and Bud Goodall's first edict of creative writing but would also be cathartic for me, as it has been for so many other cancer survivors—and some non-survivors. But life kept happening, and I kept writing, and now what began as a scattered set of personal musings has blossomed into a full-fledged saga of self-discovery. My tale holds a few surprises, and I won't give them away here, although I do want to talk a bit about the general trajectory of the story.

Echoing Robert M. Pirsig's charge in *Zen and the Art of Motorcycle Maintenance*, this narrative is my own quest for living a high quality life, both personally and professionally. At the outset, like many academicians, my personal and professional lives had become so estranged from one another that I wasn't living very productively in either one. But when I contracted cancer, clearly personal, I began to learn some lessons in survival that carried over into my life as a college professor, a place where I badly needed a new set of survival skills. What I learned (rediscovered, really) was to enact a persona I call the trickster, a rule-bending, humor-laced outsider who contests rigid organizational rules without threatening the people who uphold them. Armed with that persona, I began to write those two disparate parts of my life back together and, by so doing, discovered how to live better in both realms.

In broad strokes this story begins early, with my parents, revealing how I learned an embryonic form of the trickster relating to them, used it to good advantage during my childhood and adolescence, forgot it in favor of sheep-like dependence or wolf-like aggression in graduate school and as a young professor, rediscovered it through my cancer experiences with health care providers, and finally reframed it for my future life in academia. This is more than just a "Whitman Sampler" overview. I am offering a way for you to rethink and re-feel some of your own personal/professional life divisions and, perhaps, discover new ways to overcome them. That's what any good story tries to do.

Because I speak of real people, and not always kindly, I have changed some names to protect the not-so-innocent. I've used pseudonyms for all medical practitioners, all students, and most of my academic colleagues. I've kept proper names for family members, good friends, and a few colleagues who were instrumental to my professional development. In a few cases I created composite characters and situations in order to condense a series of events into one hypothetical episode. I have not, however, changed the name of my beloved cat. Mollie is Mollie, even if she sues me over what I say about her here.

I also want to thank some people who've been with me, in person and/or in spirit, throughout this odyssey. First and foremost, my eternal love to Janice Hocker Rushing, spouse, co-author, lifelong friend, and soulmate, "without whom—not," to steal a line from someone whose name, but not whose sentiment, I've long forgotten. Words cannot express the depth of my feelings toward Janice—although I'll try from time to time in what follows. Janice's sister Joyce Hocker, brother Edward Hocker, and brother-in-law Gary Hawk have been with me for the duration. Although none plays a central role in my story, all three have always been central to my life and have guided what I say here more than they know. I also want to thank my son, Mark Andrew Frentz, who, like Joyce, Ed, and Gary, gets little onstage time in this drama, but whose presence, love, and support I've felt throughout. Mark selflessly tracked down obscure addresses needed for permissions, took the picture that gives this old trickster a visual reality, and made endless CDs and hard copies of earlier versions of this story so that I could keep track of where I'd been and where I was going. I owe several lifetimes of gratitude to Gale Young, one of Janice's closest friends, and someone with whom I've "walked that lonesome valley," thereby refuting the old hymn that says you have to walk it by yourself. Carolyn Ellis' endless patience and wise guidance (she must have endured four or five versions of this thing) spurred me on to completion. And her partner in crime and life, Art Bochner, pressed me to make better that which I was trying to complete. So Art and Carolyn, thanks for everything. Without the confidence of Left Coast Press editor Mitch Allen this story would be a scrambled set of personal ruminations languishing on a shelf or in cyberspace. And finally, a tip-of-the-hat to Sally Brown, world-class indexer. I tried to index a book once—and almost ate my gun in the process. Happily, Sally has saved me from either fate.

Thomas S. Frentz, 2007

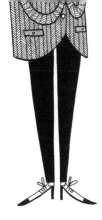

CHAPTER 1

The Call

> The call rings up the curtain, always, on a mystery of transfiguration—a rite, or moment, of spiritual passage, which, when complete, amounts to a dying and a birth.
>
> Joseph Campbell
> *The Hero with a Thousand Faces*

I feel a numbness in the right side of my groin where two lymph nodes resided until yesterday. No pain, just a slight tightness and a pulling sensation. I'm at home waiting for the pathology report and it's getting late. I try to be upbeat. After all, just two days ago the doctor told my wife Janice that the nodes were badly infected and that made it less likely they would be malignant. Being in recovery at the time, I didn't press what seems, in retrospect, to be a rather tortured logic. But now I wish somebody would have pressed. The phone rings at 4:16. I lift the receiver with as much calm as I can muster while Janice quietly listens on the extension.

"Mr. Frentz?" comes a pleasant, disembodied voice.

"Yes," I answer, not sounding like me.

"Just a second. Dr. Logan wants to talk to you," the voice continues.

Damn! I know instantly that this is not good. Part of the unwritten medical protocol here is that receptionists and nurses give good news, doctors bad. I hear another receiver click, then a more authoritative voice.

"Mr. Frentz, this is Dr. Logan. Your pathology report just came in, and you have squamous cell carcinoma in your lymph nodes. Now, this is very surprising because . . . ."

I don't hear anything after the "because," because I'm obsessively trying to spell "squamous" on the yellow legal pad in front of me. I try "squeamish," "screamish," and even "squidish" before checking back in.

"Is this life-threatening?" I ask, knowing the answer even before I hear it.

"Yes, it can be," he affirms deliberately, "but our more immediate concern is that this form of cancer does not originate in the lymph system, and that means that it's moved there from somewhere else. What we need to do is get you in for some tests and see if we can locate the primary source so that we can begin treating it."

This is where my story begins. No, actually it begins much earlier. This is only where I begin to learn how to tell it.

I've read a lot since "the call" about how people first react to being diagnosed with cancer. The accounts vary, of course, but the feelings usually don't: anger, fear, disbelief. I didn't feel any of those things at first. I felt, rather, as if this was the fulfillment of some dark destiny although I know that, technically, destiny is not a feeling. My mother died at 51 of lung cancer and my father at 65 of lymph node cancer (more of this later). I'm now 61, and, genetically speaking, a two-time loser. If I make it to 65 or beyond, I will have outlived both my parents. But because I now have "their" disease, I feel somehow empowered to retell the story that they wrote, in part, for me many years ago. I feel some urgency as well.

This empowerment, compulsion really, arose because cancer shattered the narrative coherence of my life. I am not alone here, for we all experience from time to time life-altering events that throw our well-ordered worlds into turbulent chaos. For Art Bochner, it was hearing of his father's sudden death while attending a communication convention ("Time"); for Arthur Frank, it was being diagnosed with testicular cancer less than a year after recovering from a heart attack; for Carolyn Ellis, it was the shock of her brother's sudden death in a plane crash ("Survivors"); for Lyle Crawford, it was the horror of seeing a friend being killed by an alligator. Life-disrupting experiences come in all shapes and sizes: the end of a long-term relationship, the loss of a job, the pressure of an unplanned pregnancy, the agony of an abortion, the recklessness of a romantic interlude, the uprootedness of job-related moves, the discovery of a life-threatening illness, the impending fear of madness, and so on. The events are not new—but crafting a new narrative order out of the chaos they produce can be.

On one level, this journey charts the relationship between my personal and professional selves. In many ways, it's analogous to the one Art Bochner tells about the sudden death of his father. That trauma pushed Art to examine the disjunctions between his personal and professional lives. In the process, he discovered how, through narrative, he could begin to write back together those two disparate strands of his own divided existence. Similarly, my cancer directs me to look back at the same two plotlines in my life. Because I have more time (I hope) and more space than Art had in his journal article, I have the luxury of going back a little further and looking around a bit longer. In many ways, the story I tell here is an extension and elaboration of Art's work, but I want to go about it a bit differently. I want to link my professional life with the rationality that defines all of life in the university and in the medical profession, my personal life with all those sentient feelings and bodily desires that augment and sometimes override my thinking processes in those two places, and the fusion of the personal and professional with a third element, the recovery of something called Quality. Like Art, I think that fusion entails seeing the totality of life as an unfolding narrative, but I would add that the story must itself be told with Quality or it will do little more than re-inscribe the disjunction.

What Art has done and what I am doing tie directly into a larger, ongoing set of self-reflexive stories about life in the academy. To be sure, not all these tales are motivated by life-threatening traumas, but most tell of how an academic life diminishes life in general, and almost all include moments of emotional emptiness, lost dreams, repressed angers, unfulfilled desires— what Art has called "institutional depression" ("Time"). I'll never forget the first time I read John Rodden's "Field of Dreams." John was one of the first to see how the corporate mentality surrounding academic publishing had impoverished his life. Here is his stunning moment of self-realization:

> Yes, I realized, I had become rather proficient at the academic game. But had my sense of wholeness and my nonacademic gifts paid the price? The profession so strongly approved of the imbalance that I had managed not to spot the signs of atrophy, not to notice the partial man in the mirror. Professional approval had quelled the still, small voice inside me that murmured: *This is not all of you.* (120)

"This is not all of you." And this is not all of me either. I am more than the person scripted by my parents and more than the one acculturated by my profession. It's high time I figured out who my very own *other* is. I know that it's taken me 61 years and the onset of cancer to stumble upon his existence, but I guess I'm just a slow learner.

I spoke earlier of Quality as the way to integrate our professional and personal selves. It's time to explore that term just a bit. In 1975 the paperback version of Robert M. Pirsig's celebrated odyssey of self-discovery, *Zen and the Art of Motorcycle Maintenance*, exploded on the American public. As far as I know, *Zen* is the only bestselling book about rhetoric ever written, and, I might add, one written as an autoethnography, although Pirsig never used that term. Like most beleaguered rhetorical scholars in the 1970s, and like millions of others in all walks of life, I was enchanted by this strange and mesmerizing story of spirit and cycles. Unlike most, I never forgot it. I came to believe that living a high Quality life, professionally and personally, was the most important, yet difficult, task I could ever achieve, and I've pursued it, in fits and starts, ever since. This book recounts one part of my continual quest for Quality.

In Pirsig's novel, a father and son take a motorcycle trip across the American Northwest. As they travel, the father begins to recover the shadowy outlines of a former self he calls Phaedrus (from Plato's celebrated dialogue of the same name), a solitary genius who went mad pursuing Quality, a Zen-like pre-intellectual apprehension of value. Quality, as Phaedrus came to understand it, answered the question "What is best in life?" (8). It is neither some mysterious element within objects nor some equally mysterious preference within subjects. Quality is a dynamic, immediate vision of value that occurs in that nanosecond *before* the world gets all chopped up into subjects and objects. For example, the very best things you'll read here, those with the highest Quality, I will write when the writer and the story are totally undifferentiated. In these rare moments, I am not the subject-who-writes, the story is not the narrative-being-written, but they are one and the same and grow out of the Quality event. Looked at in this way, Quality is not hard to understand. It is really captured in the expression "losing ourselves in our work." It's what happens whenever we care passionately and completely about what we are doing, whether what we are doing involves repairing an old motorcycle, programming a computer, or telling a story about university life.

What makes Quality so hard to grasp today is that it has been destroyed and replaced by rationality and its technological offshoots. Here's how Pirsig thinks it all came about. In his search for the origins of Quality, the journey of Pirsig's Phaedrus takes him all the way back to classical antiquity, where he finds Quality being taught as rhetoric by, of all people, the sophists, for whom it was understood as *aretê*, overall excellence in living (336–41). But Quality, like rhetoric itself and the sophists who taught it, fell victim to the relentless juggernaut of Plato's dialectic, a rational method of inquiry that reduced Quality to an idea, defined the idea, sliced it up into parts, and then discarded the parts as the mere debris of emotional expression and public opinion (374). Pirsig recounts the magnitude of this loss:

> And the bones of the sophists long ago turned to dust and what they said turned to dust with them and the dust was buried under the rubble of declining Athens through its fall. Through the decline and death of ancient Rome and Byzantium and the Ottoman Empire and the modern states—buried so deep and with such ceremoniousness and such unction and such evil that only a madman centuries later could discover the clues needed to uncover them, and see with horror what had been done . . . (376)

What had been done was to fashion a way of living—an entire worldview, really—known as Western civilization, that deified reason as the Godhead of goodness. But sometimes what is reasonable just isn't any good, and until recently that little secret got lost in the shuffle.

In modern times, Phaedrus found reason most firmly spiritualized within the academy, which he called, appropriately enough, the "Church of Reason." But this academic church, Phaedrus also discovered, was a low quality place of worship where professors burn out, imitation stands in for creativity, and grades are taken as signs of learning. Clearly, here is an early vision of what Art would later call "institutional depression" ("Time" 433). Extending the spiritual allegory, Phaedrus noticed that, as churches, universities house three kinds of animals. There are shepherds, those professors and administrators who reproduce the church's rational structures; sheep, those students who learn and abide by the church's rules; and, from time to time, a wolf that tries to destroy structures in the name of Quality. As Phaedrus learns, wolves never destroy churches but churches do destroy wolves.

I am neither arrogant nor foolish enough to position my own story here as a sequel to Pirsig's remarkable work. But along the way I do discover another animal, the Coyote/Trickster, that might have kept his Phaedrus sane and even helped in his pursuit of Quality. Coyote/Trickster is not quite a wolf, not really a shepherd, but rather a creature with the potential to disrupt church structures and steal back a modicum of Quality without ever threatening rational foundations. Echoing Plato's moral imperative that we become better people by remembering what our souls once knew but forgot when they became embodied in human form, my own tale tells of learning the wiles of the trickster early, forgetting them later, operating as a wolf instead, and then, only after repeated failures and setbacks, rediscovering the trickster. Pirsig writes, "A real understanding of Quality doesn't just serve the System [Church of Reason], or even beat or escape it. A real understanding of Quality *captures* the System, tames it, and puts it to work for one's personal use, while leaving one completely free to fulfill his inner destiny" (217). If Phaedrus had a little less wolf in him and a little more coyote—namely, a little more role distance on himself and a little more humor in life—he may have developed a fuller understanding of Quality.

Although *Zen and the Art of Motorcycle Maintenance* is my *über* text, others are important as well. I need a model for the rational structure of the Church of Reason—both the academic and medical versions—and, while many come to mind, I gravitate toward the one crafted by anthropologist Victor Turner because it coincides with my own experiences in both places. Turner identifies two basic forms of human relatedness, *structure*, which is hierarchical and based upon specialization, division, and exclusion (the Church of Reason), and *communitas*, which is egalitarian and grounded in identification and inclusion (96). This depicts a dialectical tension between these two such that structure attempts to repress communitas, while communitas tries to undermine structure. But for Turner, *both* structure and communitas are essential to a full social life because, while too much structure stifles individual creativity, too much communitas negates collective effectiveness. Infuriating Marxists everywhere, Turner insists that structure dominates all collectivities, and those temporary unstable periods of communitas, when they occur, function only to soften, realign, and renew structure so that it might again operate more humanely. Turner also speaks of *liminality*, a never-never land halfway between structure and communitas. Transitions more than states, liminal rituals allow shepherds to remember what it was like to be sheep, and sheep to anticipate what it will be like to become shepherds (97). There are no wolves in Victor Turner's world. Wolves are in the business of deconstructing structure, not reconstructing it through communitas.

But *canis latrans*, Wily E. Coyote, while not explicitly in Turner's world either, does his best work within liminality. This mythological character, an archetype really, lives to deflate all structures. The trickster is that "creative idiot . . . wise fool, the gray-haired baby, the cross-dresser, the speaker of sacred profanities . . . Trickster is the mythic embodiment of ambiguity and ambivalence, doubleness and duplicity, contradiction and paradox" (Hyde 7). A shape-shifter who appears in various cultures as a coyote, raven, or even a spider, she/he traffics in laughter, humor, and irony (Radin x). "You and I know when to speak and when to hold the tongue," Hyde reminds us, "but Old Man Coyote doesn't. He has no tact. They're all the same, these tricksters; they have no shame and so have no silence" (153).

Tricksters are more than mischievous misfits. Like Prometheus and Hermes, "tricksters are regularly honored as the creators of culture. They are imagined not only to have stolen certain essential goods from heaven and given them to the races, but to have gone on and helped shape the world so as to make it hospitable for human life" (Hyde 8). In their best moments, tricksters reveal ways of living that excite others to thought and action (Turner 128–29). As such, they are rhetors in the classical sense, instructing, cajoling, and challenging others to live a more humane existence.

The story I'm about to tell unfolds as a personal narrative. In ethnographic literature, personal narratives are called lots of other things as well (Ellis and Bochner 739). In social science circles, they're often dismissed as "me-search" by those seemingly terrified by the possibility that scientific knowledge might be more subjectively constructed than objectively discovered (to invoke an opposition that I'll challenge throughout). But I'm more interested in what these stories do than in what they are called. Bud Goodall says that personal narratives are "shaped out of a writer's personal experiences within a culture and addressed to academic and public audiences" (9). More radically, they collapse an entire array of binary oppositions that have traditionally given "method" its meaning in academia, the more controversial of these being, fact/fiction, subjective/objective, art/science, reason/emotion. Personal narratives are less concerned with building theory, refining method, or interrogating texts (although they may do all of those things from time to time) than they are with persuading readers to reflect upon their own lives. "But isn't that what engaging literature already does?" someone always asks about here. Exactly. Multiple functions for scholarship often occur when binary oppositions implode. Personal narratives employ literary conventions and rhetorical strategies to induce readers to revisit their lives retrospectively (9). I have written numerous personal narratives to acquaintances and friends, but only a few recent pieces are part of my published scholarship in Communication—except, well, maybe that ribald letter that got printed ages ago in *Penthouse* Forum. But that's a trickster tale for another time.

I'm writing for anyone whose "church life," either within a university or within some corporate institution, is empty and low in quality, but who still holds out hope that there are better ways to live within these cultural sanctuaries. As Pirsig constantly reminds us, Quality is not something we're just "born with" (although we are born with it), not some intuitive "knack" that some have and others don't, but rather a very practical way of relating to the world in which we live. This book is about how a trickster seeks that Quality through relating to the world in which *he* lives. I begin with several formative experiences with my parents, the first church, because that's where I first learned how to be a sheep, a wolf, and a coyote. I then move to a few lighter trickster-ish moments, just to remind myself of what I had forgotten. I also re-live a few of my worst academic moments to illustrate the self-destructiveness of the wolf's rage. With all three voices introduced, I dwell on a few details of my relationships with cancer specialists, because in those often-frightening relational episodes I rediscovered some of those lost trickster skills. With more than a little fear and loathing, I discuss some of my professional relationships to show how difficult the changes I want to make really are. For four years I didn't know how to end this book. Then, in late 2003, the ending was forced upon me with tragic suddenness.

Although I now know where this book will end, I have no idea where I will end. Life, at least my life, isn't quite that predictable or certain. I remember asking my brother-in-law, Gary Hawk, if he ever began a poem without knowing where it would end. "Oh," he replied with great joy, "I do that all the time. *That's* why I write!" I'll speak in a variety of voices—coyote, wolf, sheep, shepherd—and sometimes combinations of the four. However, as I've learned about this kind of writing, I don't always know or command the particular voice I'm using until I reflect back upon it (Richardson 2000). One thing I do know: The life of the mind in the churches of reason does not have to entail the death of the soul for those who worship there, although it can and often does. But if Quality was once buried in the ashes of antiquity, it can be exhumed again when the time is right. The time was right in 1975; I think it may be right again today.

CHAPTER 2

Women's Ways

To nourish and protect, to keep warm and hold fast—these are the
functions in which the elementary character of the feminine operates
in relation to the child, and here again this relation is the basis of the
woman's own transformation.

> Erich Neumann
> *The Great Mother:*
> *An Analysis of the Archetype*

A spring breeze cooled my back as we headed down the hall toward my room.
Her fingers curled around my hand. I shivered as my arm nudged her hip,
the musky warmth exciting and close. Quietly, we entered the dark bedroom,
save for a pale reflection from a dim hall light. The cool sheets comforted as
she sat next to me. Lying back, I felt her hand stroke my forehead. Through
dreamy, half-closed eyes, I caught her profile—slender, ultra-feminine. Slowly,
she leaned over me, her warm mouth lightly brushing my cheek. I flushed,
my body tightened. Her lips paused, sensed something—a quick kiss, quite
chaste, something more, something less—and then she sat up quickly. Almost
embarrassed, she stood hurriedly, began to say something, seemed to think
better of it, and then moved to the door of my room, the hall light again fram-
ing her body.

"Good night, Tom," she whispered huskily.

"Good night, Jo," I murmured back.

I watched her silhouette, the soft backlight illuminating a dancer's body
through her thin summer dress. As the door closed, my mind opened.

I imagine an icy February night where I am slowly picking my way through a frozen cornfield. Somewhere near the middle, I pause, drop to my knees, and begin looking for something. Yes, there it is, a tiny flash of silver beneath the dark earth. The zipper, right where it should be. I slowly unzip the top of the ground; bright, warm light floods the field. "Too bright," I worry, "someone might see." I quickly burrow into the opening and zip out the light. Here, beneath this field of dreams, I enter a tiny room filled with wonderful fantasies. I'm safely alone now.

Back in my bed, I tugged my mattress pad into a raised rib. With trembling anticipation, I pulled down my big-boy underpants. Then slowly I began to wiggle back and forth across the ridged pad, each movement sending erotic tremors through me as I became lost in innocent delight.

Suddenly a blinding light! My bedroom door flew open, slamming against the wall. Mind and body collided before the brute reality of her presence. I saw her clearly, looming over me, shaking with rage, a horrific image of the Medusa herself.

"Stop that right now, you filthy little sonofabitch!" she screamed in my face. "Don't you ever let me catch you doing that again, *ever*, you perverted bastard!"

She spun around, stormed out, and slammed the door behind her. The room shook from her rage. I shook too. I drew the sheets up over my head and curled into a tight little ball. Tears moistened the sheets, chills wracked my body, and sleep never came. But the questions did: What did I do wrong? Why was she so furious? Had I lost her love forever? Could I ever win it back, and, if so, at what cost?

In mythic terms, this is a classic Great Mother drama in which irons from my mother's personal demons sear me with a brand for living: Sex and love are mutually exclusive. If I want the intimacy of a woman's love, I must sacrifice any desire for sexual pleasure. In that one eternal now, she instilled this age-old lesson. I learned it well, internalized it deeply, and never forgot it. As an adult, it played out in projected forms as manhood issues. I was four at the time.

I don't want to leave things here for that would be really unfair to my mother. She was far more than the child-devouring monster I've sketched above. She also taught me that to love meant to give selflessly.

It was 10:15 A.M. and I was home from second grade (again), resting in their double bed.

"Jo, my ears still hurt," I complained. I always called my parents by their first names, Jo and Ted. I'm not sure why, but I think it's because I could relate to them more as people and less as parents. They didn't seem to mind. This first-name strategy is something I continued as an adult whenever I felt estranged from people by status differences.

"I know, honey, but these drops are the best we can do right now."

"But they don't help," I whimpered.

She sighed slowly, glanced out the window toward the lake for awhile, drifting apparently, and then, almost as if she'd solved a small mystery she'd been working out in her mind, she smiled.

"Lie back, on your side."

"Like this?"

"That's fine."

I felt her closeness. With measured deliberation, she lit a Kool. I watched her tilt her head back and inhale deeply. Then, cupping my head in her hands and placing her mouth over my ear, she slowly exhaled, blowing the lung-warmed smoke deep inside my head. She did this over and over—first one ear, then the other—until the cigarette burned her fingers. She lit another and did it again. Then again. Miraculously, the pain subsided. This was her healing touch to me, but there was a tragic irony at work here as well. Neither of us could have known that the smoke warmed by her lungs to cool my pain would, over time, destroy those very lungs.

I've now read and reread these two vignettes about my mother. At first I was reasonably content with them, certain that they provided an accurate portrait of our relationship. But the more I read, the less content I became. Something of consequence was missing but I didn't have a clue what it might be. So I took a page from Carolyn Ellis' description of sociological introspection ("Sociological"), gathered up some old photo albums, and pored over images of my mother and me at varying stages of our lives. There I am at two, chubby with curly locks, looking up adoringly at my mother. There she is, slim and mysterious, with curly locks of her own, looking down adoringly at me. But then there I am at eight, thinned out with a buzz cut, again looking at my mother—but how?—imploringly, questioningly. She is still looking at me, but her gaze is different, more distant, seemingly distracted by something.

At first, I didn't make too much of this; mothers and sons are supposed to separate as sons gain an independent sense of self. But this felt different, and now I think I know why. As I matured, my mother pulled away from me emotionally much more than is typical. Distraught over the loss, I was willing to do *anything* to get her back, even if that meant remaining a dependent infant. I now believe she saw through my ruse because she never again gave me what I so desired. I deeply resented regressing in order to wheedle her love, which shouldn't have been age-specific in the first place. In these reflections on faded black-and-white snapshots, I catch my first glimpse of the sheep I thought I had to remain for my mother, as well as the wolf I thought I needed to be to escape her clutches.

Fortunately for me, my mother wasn't my only mother. Her older sister Hilda gave me the very thing my mother withdrew early on: unconditional love. I both devoured Hilda's love and punished her for giving it, because it should have been given by my mother, not my aunt. But Hilda brought forth something new as well. Hilda nurtured, to a fault, my embryonic trickster. Long before *Harold and Maude* became a cinematic model for comedic mother/son perversity, I was playing some of that out with Hilda. I would cover my wrists in catsup, hide in one of her dresser drawers, and then, just as she walked in, let a catsup-dripping wrist drop out of the drawer. I sometimes put red food coloring in my bath water and then screamed that something was terribly wrong with me. We would play Indian, always on the hottest summer days, and I would force her, my "squaw," to sit in some stifling, godforsaken pup tent for hours while I, her "brave," was out "hunting game." Hilda was the most accepting, uncritical, kindest person I ever knew. When I was much older, I used to say, half seriously, that I could tie a tourniquet around my arm and say, "Hilda! Here, hold this while I shoot up!" and she'd just concentrate and hold it. Hilda modeled unselfish love. Almost every day she denied herself so that I might be happy. Hers has always been the most profound expression of mother love that I know. I was a very good student.

Hilda taught me far more than how to give. She was one of a kind, a genuine eccentric, and an independent woman who chose to live her life as few women had the courage to do at that time. Although stunningly beautiful, she never married and, as far as I knew, had only one serious relationship, with a self-destructive alcoholic. When I used to tease her about this, and I did that a lot, she would only wink and ask whimsically, "Oh Tom, whatever would I do with a man?" Still, she seemed totally happy and fulfilled, which suggested to me that happiness was not necessarily dependent upon relational intimacy. Hilda was a liberal Democrat in a conservative Republican enclave of Wisconsin and an active member of her teacher's union in Illinois. She never discussed her politics, but never wavered from them either. She taught me the rush of being a principled outsider. She also taught second grade in Oak Park, Illinois for 48 years. Over the course of those years, she instructed many children of Chicago's most notorious gangsters. She never spoke harshly of them. "The most polite, highly motivated children I ever taught," she used to tell me, "were children of the Sicilian crime lords. They always had a profound respect for teachers." During the Great Depression, when most teachers in Illinois were paid in vouchers, those in Oak Park were paid with crisp $100 bills. "Gang money," she chuckled. She told of having lunch in the Pump Room of the Palmer House with two of her colleagues one Sunday when their waiter brought them a $100 bottle of wine. "Compliments of Mr. Capone," he told her quietly, nodding towards a closed door leading to a private dining area. The "bad guys," I learned, weren't always bad and the "good guys," I would learn later, weren't always good.

Hilda loved teaching, was superb at it, and instilled in me the value of education and the wonders of an imaginative mind. She read to me constantly. I put her through the entire *Black Stallion* series and everything Albert Peyson Terhune ever wrote about collies. I would lose myself in her words and live in the images they brought forth. She encouraged me to collect butterflies, and I got so good at it that I won three blue ribbons at the Winnebago County Fair. She taught me how to spool knit, from which I spun an endless variety of hot pads and doilies that graced our tables. Because she listened so intently to everything I had to say, and made me feel important for saying it, I learned how to listen intently to what others had to say, hoping that I could make them feel good too. Hilda died quietly of natural causes at 93. I think about her often.

For my first nine years, I was socialized primarily by these two women, my mother and my aunt. Outwardly, I developed a feminine persona and came to see the world and to feel about people from that perspective. In both appearance and inner demeanor I was becoming, as Robert Bly would put it years later, a "soft man" with a gentle, caring, self-protective view of myself (2). In Pirsig's metaphor, I learned how to act like a sheep, dependent upon my two shepherdesses for almost everything I desired.

Soft men, Bly warned, lack energy, a certain fierceness (3). That was not my problem. I already had an overabundance of fierceness, a wolf nature, rooted in unconscious rage at my mother, but acted out more lightly in my coyote interludes with Hilda. Because I learned to feel from my mother and

Hilda, I absorbed their emotional attitudes toward my father, and men in general. Most mothers probably craft cute little euphemisms for their children's bowel movements. My mother's went like this: "Why don't you go make a man?" I remained innocent of the masculine loathing in that expression until my mid-fifties.

I now think that the "man" my mother asked me to flush down the toilet was none other than my father. I believe she pushed me away emotionally because she deeply feared I would eventually turn into my dad. Or, having escaped that, at least into an adult male, which would have been equally odious to her. I see now that my mother had no love for men, although I have no clue where this originated. Still ambivalent about my nascent wolf potential, I had only to look at my father to see it actualized in all its charismatic, self-destructive clarity. And by nine, as an only child, I was more than ready for some charismatic, self-destructive clarity.

CHAPTER 3

Life with Father

I've done . . . questionable things.
Roy Batty
Blade Runner

"He comes with me today."

It was a pretty ordinary Saturday morning. My dad and I were having breakfast. I was perched at our kitchen table nibbling Cheerios and sipping orange juice, while he sat nervously on the edge of his bed, washing down a shot of brandy with a bottle of Chief Oshkosh beer, and drawing deeply on an unfiltered Camel. I was ten, he was a little older.

I was scared shitless of my father. Partly, that was because I experienced him emotionally through my mother's eyes, but more viscerally it was because my father was one scary sonofabitch. He wasn't very imposing physically, only 5'5" and about 140 pounds. Every morning he used to slick his hair back with Vaseline Hair Tonic. Every night, he wore a hair net to train it to part like Cary Grant's. He dressed impeccably at work, fairly peccably when not. Most who met him were instantly turned on or off by his volatility. I remember him as a composite of James Cagney in *White Heat* and Robert DeNiro in *Cape Fear*, although he looked more like a miniature Robert Mitchum.

My father was a practical joker. He was not a trickster, at least not in the mythic sense that I previewed earlier, because his pranks seldom disrupted the structures in his life. But they did have a wolfish edge to them. I remember how he used to clutter our home with novelty toys. My personal favorite was an eight-inch plastic donkey, which adorned the coffee table in our living room. My father filled this donkey's hollow belly with dark brown cigarettes.

Whenever some unsuspecting guest would ask "Could I bum a cigarette?" my father would cheerfully say "Sure," press the donkey's tail, up it would go, and then, right before our horrified guests' eyes, a nice, brown cigarette would slowly slide out of the ass's ass. Not everybody lit up.

Then there were his annual bank parties. Because my dad was vice president of a local bank, most everyone had to show up. Thinking back on them today, I suspect they must have been absolute horrors for young female employees. My father would spend weeks ahead of time jerry-rigging our house. His favorite was the tiny microphone he taped behind the toilet seat in the guest bathroom. Whenever some unsuspecting young woman sought refuge there, my father would tiptoe up to the bathroom door, get his camera ready, and, if he had timed things right, activate a tape that would blast through the microphone, "Hey, hey, hey! Hold it lady! Can't you see I'm painting down here?" More often than not, a hysterical woman would bolt from the bathroom half-dressed and screaming—into the waiting lens of my father's camera. He just loved that sort of thing.

I remember Edie and the Cobra. In 1963, after a long series of correspondences with the rogue auto maker Carroll Shelby, my father conned Shelby into selling him, apparently against Shelby's better judgment (or so it says in one of his letters), a 289 Shelby Cobra. For the uninitiated, this car—a glorified racecar, really—was an unassuming, two-seat roadster that looked a bit like today's Mazda Miata. But Cobras were not Miatas. With an all-aluminum body it weighed slightly under 2000 pounds, and with its souped-up Ford 289 engine block with eight Weber carburetors under the hood (trust me on this stuff), this baby could fly. If my dad hit all the shifts right (a rarity, admittedly), it would go from 0 to 60 in 4.1 seconds. As far as I know, he only lost one drag race in his life, to an Indian motorcycle. He should have known better.

Edie was his main traveling companion. He bought her from a local department store. She was a mannequin, and quite fetching as I recall. I remember coming home one afternoon to see my dad painting Edie's breasts, so that she might appear more anatomically correct. His real rush, however, was to warm up the Cobra, detach Edie's torso from the rest of her, prop her securely in the front seat, wearing nothing but a smile and a blonde wig, and then slowly drive through town. Typically, these junkets would last between 15 and 20 minutes before the local police would pull him over and cite him for disturbing the peace. "This is my piece," he would say with sexist delight, "go disturb your own." They busted him a few times, but eventually they reached a compromise. If my dad would clothe Edie in *something* (a see-through white nightie became his wrap of choice), they'd allow him to drive her around town in his fast little car. I thought this was just wonderful.

"Where're you taking him?" my mother asked my father trying to sound calm but failing.

"The Silver Crest," came his laconic reply.

Now *that* sure got my attention. Maybe he didn't think I was a little sissy pants after all. The Silver Crest was a reasonably seedy bar, my dad's home away from home every Saturday and Sunday from 10 o'clock to 5:30, when he would head home, none too steadily, for dinner. For the seven-and-a-half hours in between, he would drink with his cronies, play a game of dice he invented called "Shit," lament about what insensitive bitches wives were, and relive exploits from hunting seasons.

Boys don't just "grow" into men. They must be gradually eased into these mature wonders through various rites (or wrongs) of initiation. Mine had a generational precedent. My father's mother dressed him in rich, blue satin dresses (I have the pictures), took him to country club teas, and stuffed him so full of girlish guile that he was well on his way to becoming an effeminate little wuss. One day his father literally jerked him out from behind his mother's apron strings, dragged his sorry little ass out of the house, took him to the very rough-hewn local riding stable (on which my grandfather held a considerable mortgage), tossed him unceremoniously into an empty stall of none-too-clean hay, and snarled at the stable owner, "Here! This is my pansy son. He's yours for two weeks. Make a man outa him or kill him!" It was "Outward Bound" before its time. Two weeks later my father-to-be emerged as a man. He quickly became an apprentice jockey, started raising general hell, and figured out, once and for all, that this masculine business was a helluva lot more fun than his mother's boorishly proper tea parties.

Having spent my first nine years with Jo and Hilda, Ted must have thought I was heading straight down the road to girldom. So, like his father before me, Ted decided to initiate me through his own rites of manhood. Rather than toss me in with the seedy set for a make-or-break two weeks, my dad took me along with him and his cronies. It didn't matter that we hung out in seedy bars, that he got progressively drunker as the day went by, that he talked about women the same way he talked about cars, guns, and boats, or even that we never talked straight about anything important. It didn't even matter that, after downing between 10 and 15 Bierley's orange drinks, I peed incessantly in bright orange. All that mattered was *my father took me with him*. He cared enough to do it himself.

A central part of my trickster character got worked out in the Silver Crest and places like it. I was never big on gag toys and practical jokes, and I would never dare do what I did to Hilda with my father's male cronies. Rather, my own style relied on verbal humor. I developed a lightening-quick wit that specialized in dark, scatological, perverse analogies usually devoid of any self-monitoring mechanisms. As I perfected this coyote persona, I earned the respect of my father and his drinking buddies by showing that I could play in their arena and, perhaps far more important, I forged an alternative self-identity not totally dependent upon the sheep voice I learned from my mother. I liked myself in these contexts, and felt I was becoming my own person, although, in truth, I was still in reaction to parental influences—my father's charismatic dominance or my mother's subtle seductiveness.

But my father had a darker side, a vicious wolfishness, and when he acted out of those shadow energies he became dangerous and self-destructive. He also became magnetically unforgettable, at least to me. As an impressionable teenager, Ted Unplugged was impossible to resist.

I was twelve years old, had been duck hunting with Ted for several years, and had already acquired some of the requisite skills. I was a good shot—actually, a *very* good shot. I knew endless variations of decoy spreads, depending upon the location of the blind and the direction of the wind. I could call divers—Redheads, Canvasbacks, and Bluebills—without using fancy-shmancy wooden calls. And I was hell-on-wheels with cripples. The only way they could escape me was to dive and drown themselves by hanging onto a weed. Even then I could usually find them and jar them loose with an oar.

We lived on the shore of Lake Winnebago. Every year, one week before the season opened, Ted and I would build a duck blind out of rocks and hay bales on the outermost point in our front yard, not more than 50 yards from our home. This was our personal rite of fall. Our point receded into Miller's Bay, and about seven houses down, at the end of the bay, lived Walter Doemel. I hated Walter Doemel, mainly because Ted hated Walter Doemel, and, I guess, because he didn't have a chin. Why Ted hated him, save for his chin, was less clear. I think it had something to do with moral principles, Ted fervently claiming to have some, and proclaiming with equal fervor that Walter did not. Walter never frequented the Silver Crest. I guess Walter was a gentleman farmer, if you didn't push the gentleman part too far. He owned a lot of undeveloped property along the lake shore, rented out some pretty disreputable homes to people of the same type, and, more to the point here, raised ducks—huge, tame, green-headed Mallards with calluses on their feet because Walter clipped their wings so they couldn't fly.

Walter, lacking in principles, had built a wire pen for his ducks out into Miller's Bay. Just before the season began, two local game wardens came over and told Ted that he couldn't hunt as long as Walter's pen was there because the tame ducks were within 500 yards of our blind and, as such, constituted live decoys, a no-no in the state of Wisconsin. Never one to be deterred by regulations when principles were at stake, Ted contacted his lawyer, who slapped an injunction on Doemel, claiming that his pen was in "open water," which it was, and that, as such, it constituted a navigational hazard, which it did. Justice was swift. On October 1 state officials served Walter with an official edict to take his pen down and relocate his ducks somewhere else on his property.

But it was now past noon on October 3, the season opened at 1 o'clock, and the pen was still there. What to do? My father knew. "Well—just fuck him then! If he won't take his goddamned pen down, I will." Ted jumped into our rowboat, pushed off, and headed into Miller's Bay. As I watched with starstruck envy, he turned and hollered back to me, "If any of those tame bastards swim into our decoys, shoot 'em!" I nodded, knowing that I could never shoot those helpless, land-locked capons with the callused feet and clipped wings. When Ted reached the pen, he tied the anchor rope around one post, rowed back out into the bay, and pulled the pen along behind him, leaving about 35 seriously overweight Mallards in a state of delirious and unexpected freedom. Much to my horror, about 20 headed straight for our decoy spread.

Hot on their heels now, Ted herded them toward our decoys. Only he was no longer alone. Walter Doemel, having witnessed the carnage being done to his pen, dashed out of his house, leaped into his own boat, and took after my dad. Walter caught him about 50 yards from our blind. I couldn't quite hear what they were saying, but I was pretty sure they weren't exchanging pleasantries. Their boats touched and I felt a *frisson* of anticipation. Their heads bobbed. Ted shook his fist at Walter; Walter shook his fist back at Ted. Suddenly, Walter stood up in his boat, grabbed an oar, and whacked Ted upside the head, knocking him clean out of his boat and into Miller's Bay. The water there was only waist deep so I knew that Ted was in no danger of drowning, although Walter's blow could have rendered that redundant. Then, like the creature from the black lagoon, Ted surfaced, grabbed his own oar, and plastered Walter flush in the back, dumping him unceremoniously into the bay. Standing there in waist-deep water, they flailed away at each other with their oars. My ex-jockey dad dripping wet was totally outmatched by Walter Doemel, who was 6'3" and weighed about 260.

It was time for the kid to lend a hand. I dashed into our house, grabbed Ted's 32-caliber automatic pistol, and headed back to our blind with malice aforethought. They were at least 50 yards away. I didn't know whether this pea-shooter would even go that far, much less kill anything. I told myself to aim high so that, even if I was just a little off, I still might hit something. I dropped to my knees, cradled the automatic in both hands, carefully aimed at a spot about 6 inches above Walter's worthless head, and squeezed off the first round. Nothing, just a metallic click. I squeezed again, harder this time. Still nothing, just another click. Furious now, I spun around, and there, not 20 feet behind me, stood my tearful mother with the loaded clip clenched tightly in her fist.

Ted needed 15 stitches under his right eye but Walter fared much worse. He lost his spleen, and his left kidney sustained permanent damage. I watched as my dad, bloody towel in hand, climbed into an ambulance, escorted by two of Oshkosh's finest. I was so proud of him. He took out a pukeface twice his size! I remember wondering at the time whether I could ever do something that dangerously physical. My mind had already repressed the idea that, if the gun had been loaded, I would have already performed my first full-fledged wolf act at the tender age of twelve. I fully intended to blow Walter Doemel's head off.

My father had allowed me to refine and expand my trickster nature, and, in Bly's terms, he also taught me how to become a "savage man," or even a "wolf man." Savage men, Bly cautions, do great damage to humankind, because, being uninitiated and alienated from most forms of social life, they pass their immaturity and anger along to their children (x). Learning to be a man from a motley collection of unstable stable hands hardly qualifies as a sacred initiation into manhood. Of course, I didn't know this back then. I only knew that there were bad people out there, and when some of them got in your face you took them out. Ted taught me some harsh lessons that I'm still struggling to overcome.

From three principal adults—my mother, my aunt, and my father—three personae began to take shape. A relational order began to emerge as well. For many years to come, I typically met people through my coyote/trickster because it was my most independent and self-protective lead. But over time, if I came to trust and like them, if I came to see them as shepherds, the trickster receded into the background, and the softer features of the sheep began to dominate those relationships. If, however, I came to distrust or dislike the way they shepherded me, well, there was always the wolf. Indeed, I almost always distrusted and disliked shepherds who had the potential to make me feel infantile. Authority figures were just mom and dad writ large. In a weird inversion of the food chain, my wolf hunted shepherds to protect my sheep. From somewhere in that twisted little animal farm, my coyote disappeared into the night.

CHAPTER 4

Burying Ghosts

When people haven't been buried right, their ghosts come back to haunt people.

Robert Pirsig
*Zen and the Art of
Motorcycle Maintenance*

I don't want to write this chapter because I don't want to relive my parents' deaths. But "want" doesn't really enter in here. In order to move beyond their influences, I need to bury them right, as the above epigraph reminds me. I'm not sure how to speak of their passing. My rediscovered trickster, while allowing some much-needed distance from them in life, feels too edgy and glib to address their deaths. So I'll speak mostly as a sheep. That's how I related to them as a child, so that may be the best way to bury them as an adult.

In 1949 my mother had a radical mastectomy for breast cancer. Back then, the procedure gave real meaning to the word *radical.* No subtlety, no cosmetic reconstruction, this was an amputation. She had follow-up radiation, way too much, because no one knew (or was saying) how badly radiation could compromise an immune system. She recovered, at least from the cancer. Follow-up tests revealed no signs of malignancy. But she never completely recovered from the loss of her breast. She disguised the radiation burns on her shoulder by wearing high-necked blouses and dresses. She hid the deep crater where her breast used to be beneath a bra with a silicone sac carefully sewn inside her left cup. As far as I know, she never showed my dad her mutilation.

But she showed me when I was about thirteen. I don't know what prompted it, but I walked in unexpectedly one morning while she was dressing. She looked up and, with quiet resolve, said "Here. You might as well see this thing." With that she dropped her nightgown to her waist. Her right breast appeared normal, although there were flecks of radiation burns on its side. Where her left breast once was, there was now only a deep, dark red indentation. Her ribs protruded against the scorched skin. "Feel," she insisted leaning forward. Through my embarrassment and discomfort, I tentatively reached out and touched the redness lightly. It didn't feel like any skin I'd ever touched before or since—more like charred parchment. We both looked away. I never looked again, literally or metaphorically.

Jo had a 15-year reprieve before cancer hit again. This time it was in her lungs and, given that she was a lifelong smoker, we probably shouldn't have been too surprised. This was "a new occurrence," her doctors told her, not a recurrence of her previous malignancy. Just bad luck, they guessed. She moved to Madison, Wisconsin, where I was finishing my undergraduate education, because Madison had the best care facilities with the latest cancer technologies. My dad flew down to see her every weekend. Her youngest sister, Lillian, moved into a motel near the hospital. I dropped in every couple of days, there in body but not soul. I've blocked most of the details of that time. I think she had surgery again. I know she had more radiation. And I know that near the end her doctors tried an experimental type of chemotherapy called 5FU. This was not the last time I would encounter this drug.

I saw my mother for the last time at my graduation ceremony on June 13, 1961. There wasn't much left of her by then. I learned later that she'd willed herself to live long enough to see me graduate. I also learned later that "someone" had probably "boosted" her prescribed morphine so that she might endure two hours of blistering sun in Camp Randall stadium. From halfway up in the bleachers, I watched as a nurse wheeled her in—frail, stark white, a turban covering her bald head. She's here for me, I remember thinking at the time, although I'm never there for her. After the ceremony, I went down to see her. I was madly in love with a beautiful married student at the time, and wanted her to meet my mom, because I thought they were so much alike. Jo smiled weakly, I kissed her lightly on her moist forehead, and she nodded toward Pat, seeming to know in that moment more than I did about replacement costs. After only a few moments, they wheeled her away. I never saw my mother alive again. At the time, I think I sensed, perhaps for the first time, that she was really dying and, in 1961, I was too afraid to experience that directly.

Jo died at 10:17 A.M. on June 29, 1961, with Lillian holding her hand. I know this because my father unplugged the clock next to her bed at that moment, wrote the date, time, and "That's all she wrote" on a piece of masking tape, covering the face of her clock with it. An industrial-strength alcoholic, he never touched another drop of liquor from that moment on. How terribly ironic, I've thought many times since, that she had to die before he had the strength to do the one thing she most wanted him to do when she was alive. I've always been wracked with guilt over my mother's death because I was just not emotionally strong enough to share in her slow, day-by-day decline. I know that I'm not the first to have avoided this kind of prolonged suffering. Years of therapy revealed that I idealized my mother in death in ways that distorted how she related to me in life. Although the reflection has helped some, I still feel that when she needed me most I wasn't there. It is a demon and I don't seem to be able to exorcise it, rationalize it away, or even lull it to sleep.

For the next eight years, I became my mother for my father, thereby preserving the relational dynamics between my mother and father while we both grieved her passing. I put my blossoming trickster persona on hold, kicked back into that earlier, more dependent sheep way of being, and took over the household duties. I bought basic foodstuffs, cooked a little, and cleaned a lot. Occasionally, transforming from sheep to shepherd, I carefully critiqued Ted for doing dumb or outrageous things, and for his inexhaustible penchant for buying expensive toys that I didn't think we needed. I learned how to control and guide him in the same indirect, manipulative ways that my mother used to control and guide him and me. It worked for a while because we had the same needs and shared the same sense of loss.

Twelve years after my mother died, Ted was diagnosed with cancer at age 61. It had invaded several lymph nodes in his throat, and although I never knew its brand name, I now wonder if it was squamous cell carcinoma, the kind that also visited me at the same age. I got an early release from the Army (where Ted told me I would "become a man") in order to begin graduate school at the University of Wisconsin. My dad had a few lymph nodes removed from his neck at Madison Regional Hospital, the same place where my mother died, and he stayed with my roommates and me while he suffered through chemotherapy. I remember him going in every week for treatment and then sleeping almost constantly for the next few days. I also wonder whether his chemo was the 5FU they gave to Jo. After his treatments ended, he was given a clean bill of health. But, being a lifelong smoker, he soon began to experience difficulty breathing. At my urging, he got it checked out. Great news, not the lung cancer we all feared, but something called emphysema. No big deal, we figured, like having a perpetually bad chest cold.

Ted returned to Oshkosh, where he retired from the bank, sold our lake home, moved into a two-bedroom apartment, took up slot car racing with a group of young hotshots, and was living a reasonably full life, or so it seemed to me, removed as I was in Madison at that time. I was finishing my doctoral work, dating a student, and on my way to becoming a full-fledged academic, about 180 degrees from a bank vice president. I hardly ever went home to see him. In his worst moments, I fear, he thought that I'd cast my lot with a group of unwashed, long-haired hippies and other political malcontents, but he never came right out and said that to me. Rather, he told me, not without some difficulty, that he was very proud of my education and career choice. He seemed genuinely relieved that, in his own words, "You won't waste your life in some goddamned bank."

I saw Ted for the last time in 1970. I married the student I had been dating, and we headed out of Wisconsin for my first academic job in California. At 8:30 P.M. on March 19, 1971, my dad died, a little over a year after I'd left Wisconsin. I was having dinner at my mother-in-law's when I got the phone call. But his death, like his life, was not as routine as the call led me to believe. His obituary reads in part, "Coroner Duane I. Moore said death was due to a self-inflicted gunshot wound." That single sentence still triggers a flood of feelings. "If I ever reach the point where life just isn't worth living, I'm not going to live it anymore," he used to tell me with conviction. Then he would add, almost as an afterthought, "I'll tell you another thing. They're never going to hook me up to some fucking machines that piss away my life savings." I'll never know whether his cancer came back, how difficult the emphysema had made his breathing, whether my absence intensified his isolation and loneliness, or some combination of all three. I do know that he died exactly as he said he would. Ted shot himself with the same 32-caliber automatic that I tried to use on Walter Doemel. I guess the damn thing works better when Jo isn't holding the clip.

I may have buried Jo and Ted here, but certainly not my feelings for them. Despite her brutal judgments of my infantile sexuality and her apparent distain for men, I loved Jo to a fault. For a long time I carried her image with me into most of my adult relationships with women, all to the detriment of those relationships. I loved my damaged father with an equal passion, modeling my professional life on his self-destructive assault on authority. That too, I was to learn, had its down side.

CHAPTER FIVE

Turning Tricks

> To the degree that other orders are linked to the way the
> body is inscribed, and to the degree that the link is sealed
> by rules of silence, the first stuttering questioning of those
> orders must always begin by breaking the seal and speaking
> about the body.
>
> Lewis Hyde
> *Trickster Makes This World:*
> *Mischief, Myth, and Art*

If I've buried my parents right, they should no longer haunt my psyche. I should be able to put my sheep back into his pen and turn my attentions to the early exploits of Wily E. Coyote. Even here, however, I speak in mixed tongues, for while the comic side of my trickster subverts authority, the darker tendencies of the wolf always lurk in the background, ever pushing for more attention. I'll give old *canis lupus* his due later. Here I want to revisit a few episodes of the fun trickster at work, not only because I really like this part of me but also because even these early comic interludes embody some thinly disguised hostility toward various authority figures. As such, these lighter times often prefigure the darker ones to come.

Let's begin with Mrs. Sergeant's second-grade class. The class darling was the lovely, platinum-haired Susie Isner. Everybody loved Susie—most of all, Susie. I loved Susie, but unlike my candy-assed peers, I intended to do something about it. We'd just returned to homeroom after recess. I studied Susie closely, biding my time, watching for an opening. She sat down at her desk, tilted her perfect head back ever so slightly, took a pearl-handled brush

43

from her bright pink plastic purse, and began brushing her buttercup locks. That was more than I could bear. So I got up, went boldly where no boy had ever gone before, bent down, and planted a big wet one squarely in the middle of Susie's blush-pink cheek.

"Thomas!" boomed Mrs. Sergeant.

"Ma'am!" I boomed back.

"Susie doesn't want your kisses." This came with an assuredness I just didn't trust.

"Why don't we let Susie decide?" I suggested as a reasonable alternative.

In these four quick lines, my fate was sealed. I was off to see the Principal. And for *what*? All right, I guess I did lean on Mrs. Sergeant a bit, threatening her face in front of the class. But for a second-grader with an active imagination and a quick mouth, this was a pretty good moment. The only sad thing was that I never found out what Susie decided. I did find out what the Principal decided; I shouldn't kiss Susie anymore. He made that pretty clear.

My junior high was called a training school because it was part of Oshkosh State Teacher's College. Most of my teachers were young graduate assistants trying to figure out what it meant to be a secondary school teacher in the state of Wisconsin. My seventh-grade English teacher was Miss Polk; that's important not only because Miss Polk was smart and fun, but also because she was the daughter of President Polk—not the old geezer who once ran the country, but an equally old geezer who currently ran the college. Vivian liked me. I always called her Vivian outside of class because I knew she was secure enough in who she was for me not to have to call her anything else.

One bright November morning we were doing vocabulary exercises. I came in late, but then I always came in late in November because I'd been duck hunting. Vivian was peeved, I could tell right off.

"Thomas," she said with a pointed intensity.

"Miss Polk," I pointed back with equal intensity.

"Construct a sentence with the word *where* in it," she commanded.

"Today Miss Polk seems to have forgotten her underwear," I fired back with a bit more bravado than was called for.

Vivian strangled back the giggles, but she was trapped and we both knew it. She couldn't let me get away with this in a classroom overflowing with adolescent hormones. Surely against her better instincts, she sent me off to see her dad. He asked what happened, so I told him. He just stared at me like I was some creature from another world. "Master Frentz, I think you should go home and think about what you did for the rest of the day," he intoned, raising Presidential condescension to an all-time high. So I went home, hunted more ducks, and never gave Vivian's underwear, or lack thereof, a second thought. Until now.

Although these early episodes foreground my trickster and background my wolf, graduate school brought the two together as an unstable hybrid. I began the MA program in Speech Communication at the University of Wisconsin in 1964. Between 1961 and 1964, I taught speech at the Army Information School in Fort Slocum, New York. Even as a lowly private, I was teaching officers how to talk. I not only loved it but I was also good at it, and knew that college teaching (I didn't know too much about the research part yet) was my professional calling. And so I got an early out from the Army, conned my way into the Speech Communication graduate program at Wisconsin (with an undergraduate GPA of 2.34, conning was my only option), and never looked back until I received my PhD in 1970. It was during graduate school that my coyote mated with my wolf.

The clearest example of this animal union happened during my PhD orals. Now, PhD orals are frightening, immensely important, sphincter-clenching ordeals. Typically, they are two-hour sessions where four or five high-powered faculty members (one of whom is your doctoral advisor) quiz you on your dissertation, the one thing, at this point in your academic career, that you know better than anybody in the world, because that's all you've been doing for the past two to three years. But, depending upon the perversity of your chairperson and the collective arrogance of the rest of your committee, they may well ask you about anything from unsplitting an infinitive on page 128 to considering a different line of work. This is also the committee's last chance to remind you that, no matter how smart you think you've become under their tutelage, you're still not as smart as they are. Shepherds are always superior to the sheep they tutor. I have some difficulty with these situations, but before unpacking this particular one, I need to introduce Fred.

Fred Williams was my doctoral advisor but he was much more than that. He was a "good shepherd," someone I came to respect and admire greatly—a surrogate father, really, or, to complete an analogy: Fred was to Ted what Hilda was to Jo. We had, as we would have to have if he were to fulfill this paternal role, an unusual professor/student relationship. He called me Brain Damage because I was not as swift with statistics as he thought I ought to be, and I called him Captain Science because I thought his exclusively empirical world-view was limiting. He didn't think I could count and I wasn't sure he could think. But Fred was the clearest writer I'd ever read and the finest lecturer I'd ever heard. I attended every class he taught, took copious notes on his teaching strategies, studied carefully how he fleshed out even the most eso-teric linguistic constructs with clear, subtle, often humorous examples, and then, later, patterned my own lecture style after his. Could anyone illustrate a phonetic homonym any more clearly than with "The sons/suns raise/rays meat/meet," or the passive construction any more playfully than with "The Queen was pleased by the flower"? I was a willing sheep to this profoundly skilled shepherd.

Fred guided me through my dissertation, an offshoot of a grant he had to study inner-city speech patterns. I did a tedious quantitative comparison of African American and Anglo children's use of some tiny grammatical distinc-tion that we all thought was terribly important back in 1970. I ran an eight-way analysis of variance (ANOVA in stat-speak) with four nested variables. I had 256 sources of variance, eight of which would probably have been statisti-cally significant by chance alone. If any comparisons were statistically signifi-cant, how could I tell whether the significance was theoretically important or simply a function of chance expectation? I even had one significant eight-way interaction. How could I possibly explain what that might mean theoretically? I knew that if anyone asked these sorts of questions, I would be in deep meth-odological doo-doo.

As was customary, Fred began by asking me to present an overview of what I had done. I was ready for this; all candidates are ready for this. It's really just a throat-clearing exercise to keep us from throwing up and/or fainting, and for the committees to think of something to say. I zipped through this, and could see that my committee was impressed. Then, as is also customary, Fred reviewed the format of the orals. Each committee member would ask some questions and others would follow up if they saw fit, until everyone was satisfied. Fred said, "I'll start." Wait a minute! Chairs don't start, they finish. I smelled a set-up.

"So," Fred commenced, "I see that on page 24 you claim that the type of comparison you want to do has never been done before. But further back, on page 14 I believe, you cite a study which has done *exactly* what you do here," he concluded with measured certainty. "So you've done little more here than to replicate what someone else has already done. And while no one could ever question the value of replication," he added with syrupy condescension, "we generally expect dissertations to be a bit more original than that." This last line was delivered with icy contempt and a look of resigned disappointment.

I was livid but not naive. I knew that Fred had forgotten more than I'd ever know about dialect differences in American English speech patterns, but I also knew that, unless he was reading his own stuff, he had a tendency to read quickly. I also knew that I was well covered on the point he had just raised.

"You stupid sonofabitch!" I began confidently. "If you'd read with your head instead of your ass, you'd have seen that on page 24 I indict the piece of shit on page 14 for not adequately operationalizing the grammatical distinction in question *and* for using a racially biased experimental design. Now there may very well be some problems with this study," I softened just a bit, "but you're gonna have to read a fuck of a lot more thoroughly than you've done here if you're gonna find them!" This one came out like a line drawn in the sand. An unadulterated wolf snarl, to be sure.

My committee was stunned—aghast really—and shifted uncomfortably in their chairs. They must have thought that this one was over before it began. Fred shifted in his own seat, allowed the rising anxiety to just hang there while he savored the moment. Then, very slowly and deliberately, he leaned back, clasped his hands behind his head, and broke into a huge grin.

"All right, BD!" he finally said triumphantly. "I knew your brain wouldn't kick in until you got down to the shit/fuck level. So now that you're down there we can begin. Lloyd, why don't you start us off?"

Although I didn't know it at the time (I was too pissed), this episode was to become very important to me. Mythically, my unmonitored outburst was more wolf than coyote. The coyote/trickster side of it only came to the fore because Fred brought it there. His strategic humor, only revealed after my snapping response, redirected and reframed the meaning of the exchange from hostile and confrontational to an in-joke commentary between two people who knew each other very well. Without Fred's shepherding guidance, I could very well have gnawed my way out of a PhD. Fred saved me then, but he wouldn't always be there to keep my wolf in check.

I now see some other things in that oral defense that I didn't see at the time. For one, my repressed anger at authority figures was intensifying. For another, in Fred's apparently careless reading of my own careful work, I enacted an early version of a self-destructiveness that would follow me throughout my academic career. I began to question my previously unshakable belief that academic shepherds were

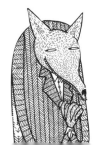

wise, knowing, and compassionate. I'd wanted to model myself after Fred, the shepherd with principles. And I suppose he did "save me" (and some embarrassment of his own) by reframing my comments as an expected response to his set-up. Be that as it may, in my oral defense I caught a reflection in Fred's admittedly comic strategizing of the same authority manipulation that I'd tried so hard to get beyond. I began to see, with considerable sadness, that the phrase "good shepherd" might well be an oxymoron. I repressed this vision for a while, anesthetizing my wolf by dressing him in sheep's clothing. But I should have known that wolves never take well to cross dressing.

CHAPTER 6

Sheep Speak

I'd guess that you're clutching the very speech. If that's
the case, please realize that though I'm very fond of you,
when we have Lysias right here, I have no intention of lending
you my ears to practice on. Come, show me!

Socrates
Phaedrus

It's unusually hot and muggy for Madison in late May. The spring 1968 semester is winding down and so am I. As a teaching assistant for the multi-section Fundamentals of Speech Communication course, I watch listlessly as the last few survivors of section 26 wearily turn in their final exams. Then there's one left. "Come on, Josh," I say to myself, "wrap it up, my man. Summer's waiting." Even here, in his last class act, Josh stays in character, making everything seem just a little bit harder and a little more tiring than I think it needs to be. With an audible sigh that's too apparent not to notice, he finally stands and trudges up to my desk. Scruffy, bearded, and sullen, Josh could have been a poster child for the dropped-out hippies of the times. My problem is, I like him a lot. He's bright, critical, playful, and often sees things that I miss. With any luck on his final exam, he'll get a "D" in Speech Communication. Not that he gives a shit one way or the other, which is another reason I like him. He's a wolf in the making.

"So Frentz," he yawns, tossing his exam across my desk. "Wanna know what's wrong with this class?"

"Of course, Josh, I *always* want to know what's wrong with this class," I yawn back in my most condescending shepherd tone.

"You take something kind of interesting, speech communication, and you just drain all the life out of it with these goddamned pseudoscientific-sounding terms. Speakers become 'encoders,' listeners are 'decoders,' talk has to be 'messages,' 'paying attention'—my personal favorite, is 'feedback'—and relationships are 'systems.' And so here I am, reasonably open to this speech shit, having to learn complex names for commonsense ideas. It's no mystery to me why your whole class mentally checks out after the first few weeks. What's with you guys, anyway?"

"Well, 'what's with us guys,' Josh, is that if we taught you what you already know in ways that you already understand, who would pay us for doing it?" I ask, not realizing at the time that I had just voiced the economic rationale for all those who try to make a science out of an art.

"Maybe nobody should," he shoots back before turning away and beaming himself back up to the *Enterprise.*

Josh had a point back there in 1968. He saw clearly what I wouldn't even catch a glimpse of for another 30 years—that communication is not some inert "thing" that you can pin down on a lab table and dissect into an array of parts. You scientize the subject, you kill the process. It's as simple as that.

Today, of course, a lot of people see what Josh and others like him saw in 1968. The vision now spreads out beyond the classroom and into our academic research. Where Josh saw how we were trying to turn the practical art of effective communication into a jargon-filled pseudoscientific practice, others are now seeing how we turn the same trick with our scholarship by taking the writer out of our writing. I particularly like Art Bochner's take on things because he not only sees his way into the problems but he also sees a way out of them. Thus, while struggling to resist the social science conventions that constrain how most chapters for disciplinary handbooks must be written, he grumbles to Carolyn Ellis, "Look at any handbook on your shelf and what you'll find is that most chapters are written in third-person, passive voice. It's as if they're written from nowhere by nobody. The conventions militate against personal and passionate writing. These books are filled with dry, distant, abstract, propositional essays" (Ellis and Bochner 734). Later in this same deliciously subversive handbook chapter, Art echoes Josh's complaints and moves beyond them:

> A text that functions as an agent of self-discovery or self-cre-
> ation, for the author as well as for those who read and engage

the text, is only threatening under a narrow definition of social inquiry, one that eschews a social science with a moral center and a heart. Why should caring and empathy be secondary to controlling and knowing? Why must academics be conditioned to believe that a text is important only to the extent it moves beyond the merely personal? . . . Why should we be ashamed if our work has therapeutic or personal value? (746)

In many ways, the story that I'm telling here attempts to honor this alternative way of doing scholarly research. But I didn't always write this way. Like most young scholars at Research I institutions, I wrote within the ideological guidelines of the social sciences (Rose). In a phrase, I wrote "sheep speak."

I've never liked sheep speak all that much—not because I couldn't do it, not because what I wrote was patently awful—but because those ironclad rules instilled by shepherds never allowed the tricksterish elements of my voice to be heard. I got to where I could do sheep speak pretty well. I'm a good critic who can uncover and spin out infinite nuances of textual meanings. I also can see underlying commonalities among seemingly disparate ideas, and this gift for metaphor allows me to generate some fairly innovative theoretical insights upon occasion. And, thanks to Fred, I can write clearly, concisely, and with a tightly wound sense of argumentative rigor. When called upon, I can chain out if/then inferences until Hell freezes over. All of these compositional skills are quite in keeping with what's expected in hardcore academic scholarship. But there are ghostwriters in my past, and I need to exorcise them from my soul, almost more than I need to cast off those outdated rules from the Enlightenment. Like most ghosts, mine are very well hidden and deeply entangled in my writing style. So, to catch them off guard, I want to sneak up on them a bit indirectly.

It was 1983 and I'd just been fired (aka: denied tenure) again (the first time having been in 1974 from that California university). This time I was asked to leave one of the more idyllic settings in the Rocky Mountains. Having already done this once, I remembered well how much fun it was to pack up and leave. The evening I received my second pink slip, I headed off to a Chinese restaurant with a few sympathetic colleagues and Larry Rosenfield, an old friend, former mentor, and co-author, who, bizarrely enough, was in town to interview for the chair vacancy in our department. After dinner, I opened my fortune cookie and read: "Avoid repetition of the same error." Too little, too late. My wolf was already peeking out of the forest. I was dressing like Waylon Jennings, inciting students against the faculty, giving bananas fellatio during faculty meetings, and prefacing all faculty meeting minutes (I was the secretary) with obscure quotations from *Moby Dick*, suggesting that the current faculty and the crew of the Pequod may well be headed for similar fates.

But my shepherd was hanging around too. After a long courtship, Janice Hocker Rushing and I were finally together in the same department, I was serving on about twenty doctoral committees, publishing regularly in prestigious forums, and teaching mass lecture classes with over five hundred student credit hours per pop. Ever the romantic, I just assumed I was so indispensable that I had more than earned the right to be a tad eccentric. Can't a good shepherd howl now and then? Apparently not.

This time the wolf in me vowed to take a few down with me. I had this nagging suspicion that all was not right with my promotion and tenure file. So I slipped into my chairperson's office late one evening and had a look. Sure enough, right there alongside the legitimate letters I knew would be there, were two I didn't know about and that shouldn't have been there. Although neither had much good to say about me, I became fixated on a single paragraph from one letter. The writer had been a visiting big deal at Wisconsin one summer when I was finishing my doctorate. Fred Williams, this visitor, and I had spent numerous evenings guzzling beer, sharing ideas, and swapping disciplinary gossip. A friend, I had thought, or, at the very least, not someone who would write nasty things about me behind my back. I don't have the letter anymore, but I can reconstruct that hateful paragraph almost word for word; it's that etched upon my soul:

> Frentz has no recognizable voice. When he writes with Rosenfield, he sounds like Rosenfield, when he writes with Farrell, he sounds like Farrell, and when he writes by himself, he doesn't sound like much of anybody. So it's hard to figure out what, if anything, he actually contributed to his published research. My own suspicion is that he has spent the better part of his career piggybacking on the superior knowledge and writing skills of his more gifted co-authors. That's hardly the mark of an emergent scholar.

Even after twenty years, the words still cut deep. What hurts most now, however, is not the condescending dismissal of my scholarship, but how unerring he was about my lack of voice. I had a scholarly voice—everyone who writes does—it's just that mine was all tamped down into sheep speak. The writer never saw this, he never knew me well enough to see much of anything, but *I* intuited it then and came to see it ever more clearly with the benefit of hindsight.

I remember how passionately I tried to rationalize away his indictment. "*No* academic scholar has 'a voice,'" I reasoned. "Real voices, interesting voices, voices anyone would want to read are prohibited by the ideological conventions of academic writing because they contaminate the objective advancement of theory, method, and knowledge." But this rationalization collapsed even as I was constructing it by the words in the very paragraph it was designed to contest. Obviously, the writer believed that at least two scholars, Farrell and Rosenfield, had "voices," even if I didn't. Not only that, but he implied that their voices actually *facilitated* their scholarship. This defense folded early.

Next, I tried the-best-defense-is-a-good-offense move. "Now wait just a minute," I thought defiantly. "I've already *done* theory, method, and knowledge, and I've done them in data-based social science pieces, humanistic theory articles, detailed critical interpretations, and even one essay that extended the logic of the scientific method." Inspired now, I basked in the warmth of my own wonderment (forgetting, I guess, that I'd been fired twice). "I'm good at it too. Almost half of my publications are lead essays (surely one quantitative sign of quality), a whole gaggle of them have been reprinted in various anthologies, I won the NCA Golden Anniversary Monograph Award for the best published article in 1976, and I even won the Best Published Article in the College of Arts & Sciences in 1978 from the very university that just fired me!" By almost any critical standard I could think of—quality or quantity—I was a successful scholar, voice or no voice, job or no job. This defense wasn't even an empty rationalization. I had *data*, for godsake. So why wasn't I buying it?

I didn't know for almost twenty years. Then, as I was reading for a seminar I was developing on ethnographic methods, I stumbled across this revelation in Anne Lamott's *Bird by Bird*. "When I was still drinking," a friend once told her, "I was a sedated monster. After I got sober, I was just a monster" (198). Finding our voice, Lamott says, forces us to quit drinking and write about our monsters rather than trying to sedate them. "When [writers] let their monsters out for a little onstage interview, it turns out that we've all done or thought the same things, that this is our lot, our condition" (198). As I thought about her words, it occurred to me that my own monsters were all those valued shepherds, some of whom I read with reverence, others with whom I wrote in awe, but all of whom had voices that dominated my own. And there is little doubt that Ted and Jo were the first two voices to have dominated my own. If I'm ever to move beyond sheep speak in my academic writing, then I'm going to have to give a few of these shepherds some onstage time to see the ways in which I depended upon them for what I wanted to say.

I begin with two samples of my single-authored research, published during a fairly productive period of my academic career. In 1985 I was hot to recover the moral potential of the classical rhetorical tradition. At that time, my principal shepherd was the highly acclaimed moral philosopher Alasdair MacIntyre and his influential book, *After Virtue: A Study in Moral Theory.* Here was a scholar who actually theorized about the very Quality that Pirsig sought and that drove my own emerging story here. But, as I read his work more closely, I discovered that MacIntyre had done himself what he accused other moral philosophers of doing, namely, combine concepts from incompatible moral traditions into a single ethical system. After showing how MacIntyre appropriated teleology from Aristotle and the quest from earlier, pre-Socratic treatises, I complete the argument:

> What MacIntrye fails to see is that a narrative quest in the
> Homeric tradition is inextricably linked to a supernatural
> *telos*—the desires and actions of the gods, as memorialized in
> poetry. As narrative quests, Homeric poetry presents the stories
> of the gods (*nomoi* or "custom laws") as normative models of the
> stories humans should live if their lives are to be characterized
> by *arête*—overall excellence. . . . By divorcing the narrative quest
> from the gods, MacIntyre has changed its meaning, and, in so
> doing, created a moral fiction of his own. When he then grafts
> that fiction onto a teleological tree, itself having been pruned
> of its theological impulse in the form of Aristotelian animism,
> the resultant bush does not exactly burn with moral authority.
> ("Rhetorical Conversation" 15)

Even after fifteen years, this is pretty good sheep speak. I still admire the so-phisticated reasoning coupled with a fairly high level of erudition that shows I can play with the shepherds. The burning bush metaphor, which in most contexts would either be dead or at least on life support, offers a nice religious tweak on an old Jesuit who seems to have lost faith in using faith in his think-ing. I'm also still fond of the recursive "watch-me-do-to-him-what-he-does-to-them" move, which shows a certain modicum of panache. Finally, when I read this passage aloud, I like how it sounds, exhibiting a well-balanced ca-dence and rhythmical flow.

But, when I focus upon the voice in this paragraph, I discover that I *sound* more like MacIntyre than like me, or, for those who know his work well, like "Mac-lite." Especially here, where I'm questioning a few moves that he makes, and should be speaking most clearly in my own voice, I'm still trying to imitate MacIntyre's unique style of philosophical argument. Some sort of "voice blending" is probably inevitable whenever someone relies extensively upon an authoritative scholar with a distinctive writing style. But, try as I might, I find no clearer trace of "me" here than I would find in those earlier social science adventures I've chosen not to revisit. I seem to have lost myself in MacIntyre's literary presence just as I once lost a younger self in my parents' physical presence. The shepherd has overwhelmed the sheep.

In reviewing subsequent work, I discovered that my shepherds came in many forms. By 1988 I was devouring everything I could find by Julia Kristeva, Luce Iriguay, Héléne Cixous, and any other female French scholar who took her Freud or Lacan straight. Armed with some formidable feminist weapons, here is my preview on how I intend to "interrogate" (that's how poststructur-alist shepherds talked back then) Umberto Eco's interminable and uncompro-mising novel *The Name of the Rose*:

> It is in the form of semiotic irruptions into the symbolic order
> that the feminine intrudes upon the patriarchy. If this is true in
> general, we should not be surprised to find it enacted in par-
> ticular within the confines of *The Name of the Rose*. By focusing
> upon the signs of the feminine in both the characters and in the
> signifying practices those characters either value or produce, we
> see a comic inversion of the historical process just summarized,
> such that the feminine semiotic "penetrates" the various patriar-
> chal texts that permeate Eco's work. ("Resurrecting" 129)

Whatever is going on here, it seems light years removed from the Apollonian heights of Alasdair MacIntyre's moral philosophy. As long as we're lingering with Lacan for a moment, I should probably acknowledge the fairly transparent psychoanalytic point that when I lose myself among the stronger, more distinctive voices of the feminist scholars introduced here, I at once reconstitute my earlier dependence upon my own mother, and, in the very same gesture, attempt to recover, through these feminist arguments, a textual form of the very sexuality my mother once tried to strip from me in infancy. Be that as it may, the more important question is, how does this feminist fragment affect my voice?

More good ewe talk here. I seem reasonably comfortable mirroring Lacanian structuralism. The metaphoric inversion of feminine meanings "penetrating" masculinized texts is, even now, a nice touch. Still, there's not much "me" to be found. In an ironic reflection of the general point of the paragraph itself, these feminist voices dominate me just as the voices of patriarchy dominate women. Even where I cautiously peek out from behind their skirts (I'm thinking of the sentence beginning "By focusing upon . . . "), my voice is heavily insulated by poststructural idioms. Although it's hard to tell from this short passage, the syntax of the entire article mimics that of Julia Kristeva and Gerda Lerner, my primary shepherds in this piece.

So much for my single-authored scholarship. What happens when I write with others? Because that poison pen letter mentions Tom Farrell as one off whom I feed, I start with a snippet from one of our co-authored pieces. In 1976 we crafted a critical framework for examining rhetorical texts from a blend of Wittgenstein's language-games and Austin's speech act theory. In a 1979 follow-up piece, we used this framework to unscramble some long-standing problems of meaning. Here is our opening gambit:

> We are intrigued by a recent tendency in both philosophic
> and scientific research to disjoin conceptions of *meaning* from
> conceptions of *communication*. Those schools of philosophy
> that assume a textual analogue for discovery make the most
> pronounced separation; as Hayden White noted: "The dispar-
> ity between speech, *lexis*, or mode of utterance, on the one
> side, and meaning, on the other, is of course a fundamental

tenet of modern Structuralist and post-Structuralist theories of the text." . . . In this essay, we suggest evidence that supports a restricted but alternative thesis: that some features of meaning are uniquely communicative. This is to say that there are aspects of meaning for some fragments of discourse that can only be uncovered by considering their functions as instances of communication. Moreover, the exploration of communicative meaning should yield important implications for scholarship in philosophy, aesthetics, and the social sciences. (215)

The academically valued conventions are still here: concise ideas, pertinent citations, and a well-crafted argument. But the voice doesn't sound like me. I would never say things like, "Those schools of philosophy that assume a textual analogue for discovery make the most pronounced separation . . ." As I reread it here, I'm not even sure I know what this sentence *means*, and this is supposed to be an article about what sentences mean. This is vintage Tom Farrell, complex, layered, careful, qualified, opaque, and very erudite.

Since we admittedly share some compositional skills, how can I be so sure that Farrell speaks here more than me? One way to find out is to compare how we sound together to how Tom sounds when he writes alone. If he sounds more different by himself than he does when we write together, then perhaps I am being too harsh on myself. Here's Tom four years later, sorting out some fairly subtle and neglected aspects of coherence common in conversation and rhetoric:

Thus it is that rhetoric, heir to a checkered history at best, has been dismissed or openly disparaged by writers ranging from MacIntyre (1981), to Ricoeur (1978), to Apel (1976). . . . Understandably, rhetoric suffers somewhat by way of contrast. More to the point of our present concern, important questions of coherence within conversation suffer as well. When conversation is seen as the principle or only avenue for attaining coherence, explaining coherence and its absence within conversation is not easy. Either questions of coherence are begged through the mythos of meaning (an intelligible content is, by communicative definition, coherent) or these questions are set aside (real discourse is distorted by the world; only free, emancipated, unconstrained social worlds allow for coherent discourse). (260)

To me, this passage sounds a lot like the one directly above. The proliferation of fairly lengthy dependent clauses, the challenges posed by a complex, embedded syntax, and the unquestioned comfort zone with the intricacies of logical entailments (begging questions, true by communicative definition, and so on), are all hallmarks of Farrell in action. To some degree, I can imitate his style of writing, but it doesn't come easily to me or flow naturally from me. I've got to work way too hard at it. The dominant voice in both snippets involving Farrell is more him than me. It seems that even the closest of shepherds, and Tom has always been that to me, speaks both for and through me.

The co-authored article with Tom Farrell comes from the 1970s, the disco era, for heaven's sake. Maybe my conclusions are dated as well. Maybe I've changed over the years, developed more of my own distinctive style, let a little trickster, or even a little wolf, slip in—or out. To check this out, I want to compare the voice in a recent co-authored work with my spouse Janice Rushing with the voice in her writing alone. Once again, if they sound alike, I haven't changed all that much, but if they sound different, then perhaps I have.

In 1999 we confronted directly the malaise of academic scholarship. Although we were novices at the time, we tried to write in a manner consistent with the argument we were making. The argument was that the sterility in academic writing stems from overvaluing metaphors of "upness" and speed, all the while repressing the realities of "downness" and repose that figure into any creative process. Mythically, the academy gives far too many awards to Apollo and far too few to Dionysus. After showing how the Greeks understood and lived through this same up/down dichotomy with creative ingenuity, we come around full circle to our own times:

> Some of us scholars think of ourselves as "artists," but we guess
> that most do not. The lines are fairly clear, not only in the divi-
> sion of our colleges into "Arts and Sciences," but more centrally
> on our annual faculty reviews, where we are to list evidence of
> "Research *or* Creative Activity." . . . But are we not all, whether
> we call ourselves artists or scientists, really Apollo's offspring,
> molding forms of knowledge out of alien mud, striving to create
> something that, if not satisfying our appetite for beauty, will at
> least outlast our own brief tenure in the academy? If so, then we
> should remember that Dionysus is the intoxicated one, and make
> time to give in to his demand for divine madness. Every person

who has ever tried to create something good, out of whatever materials, knows that one's ardor for form must, like the god, be periodically dismembered, that one must become *possessed*, just a little bit crazy, or the muses will not speak. (242)

A powerful undertone of gentle assertiveness grounds this paragraph in ways that do not ground the excerpts cited earlier. There's also a fairly radical argument at work here, tracing how unconscious, often volatile, creative forces infuse all truly inspired academic work. Finally, there's a quiet caring here—for ourselves and for those unnamed others whose work we're calling into question. I like all of these subtle sensibilities. No, better still, I *love* them, because they are so much a part of what I love about Janice as a person. They are also a large part of me, although I would express them somewhat differently. But make no mistake about it, the voice in this passage is Janice's through and through. My sentiments and values are there, but other than that, I'm pretty much along for the ride.

I turn finally to Janice writing on her own. In the late 1980s she argued how the films *Alien* and *Aliens*, far from being the paeans to feminism that some claimed, are in fact regressive narratives that split the Great Mother archetype into her Good and Terrible guises, and then pit the two against one another. As she usually does, she concludes with what we've come to call, laughingly, her "Come to Jesus" speech:

The new myth for humankind needs to be a *quest*, not a conquest; it's purpose, to *search* rather than search and destroy. Projections of an *inner other* must be withdrawn. In America, we seem to have finally dispensed with transforming the Dionysian god into an Indian (although tragically too late for the benefit of their culture). But other targets have been found, and can always be found as long as we do not wrestle with the horned demon gatekeeper inside. Only when we are ready to accept the challenge will we find what has been lost, face the Goddess in all her radiance and wrath, and decide what to do. (21)

For starters, the spiritual tone, so much in evidence above, cuts through this passage as well. The almost rhythmical contrasts, "quest/conquest," "search/ search and destroy" establish a definite antithetical cadence that's way too subtle for my tastes or abilities. And finally, here as above, there's the strong personal commitment, in marked opposition to the objective bias of the academy, to the legitimacy and the importance of the inner life as something other than a repository for scurrilous Freudian repressions. This commitment, recurring in a dizzying variety of forms like a mantra throughout her work, has become one of Janice's signature moves. As I reflect on the two passages involving Janice, I see her voice dominating both. It's a good voice—no, it's a great voice—but it's not my voice.

I want to leave these academic golden oldies now. In revisiting some of them here, I realize how dangerously close I've come to what a colleague once called "drinking your own bath water." It is clear to me how much my professional writing style, by relying so heavily on famous others or valued coauthors, produces a voice that is little more than a distant echo of shepherds I've known and sometimes loved. This autoethnographic story, the one I'm in the midst of writing right here, will, I hope, allow more of "me" to re-enter the tale. But the re-entry will be slow, and sometimes tedious. So now we've taken a look at some trickster tales and some sheep speak. Shepherds notwithstanding, there's only one animal act left in my psychic repertoire.

CHAPTER 7

Or Comes the Wolf

When a shepherd goes to kill a wolf, and takes his dog to see the sport,
he should take care to avoid mistakes. The dog has certain relationships
to the wolf the shepherd may have forgotten.

Robert M. Pirsig
Zen and the Art of
Motorcycle Maintenance

Although I've read quite a bit about the trickster, I've never seen him referred
to as a wolf. In Greek antiquity, he is Hermes; in Nigeria, he is called Eshu (for
Devil); and in most Native American traditions, he appears as a coyote (and
almost always as a male) but occasionally shape-shifts into a raven or even a
spider (Hyde). One passage on tricksters by C. G. Jung kept coming back to me.
From within his own psychological perspective, Jung speaks of conscious and
unconscious forms of the trickster. As an unconscious complex, Jung writes, the
trickster can erupt in savage, animalistic, and often self-destructive behaviors,
but if assimilated into conscious awareness and nurtured through humor, it can
become creative, spiritual, and life-affirming (*Four* 135–52). The *conscious* form
of the trickster is in keeping with both the coyote tradition in Native American
mythology and with my own singular attempts to disrupt hierarchy and question authority through comic ridicule. But that *unconscious* trickster, the one
that sometimes erupts into consciousness through savage and self-destructive
acts, seems to be an animal of a different breed.

Then I came across Scott Leonard and Michael McClure's account
of the Norse trickster, Loki. "Loki . . . may appear to be the wolfish cousin
of Coyote, but he is conspicuously less genial in nature. . . . Loki isn't fun

loving or warm; his appetites proceed not from friendly bodily urges, but from more sinister psychic cravings. . . . If Coyote embodies the creative potential of chaos and following one's impulses, Loki embodies their potential for destruction" (277–78). In this light, the wolf might very well be the appropriate canine for the unconscious, aggressive form of the trickster.

With that wolf/coyote distinction in mind, I want to return to Robert Pirsig's odyssey of self-discovery, *Zen and the Art of Motorcycle Maintenance*. On the surface, *Zen* tells of a father and son's cross-country motorcycle trip. As they travel, the father begins an oral history ("Chautauqua"), which explains his previous mental collapse, charts the technological malaise of (post)modern America, delves into social alienation in the academy, and eventually winds all the way back to classical antiquity and the struggle between the sophists (rhetoricians) and philosophers (dialecticians) over control of the Western mind. As the father's story unfolds, he begins to uncover the shadowy outlines of a former self, a brilliant, obsessive, somewhat reclusive, self-destructive personage who was psychically erased by electric shock treatment, but who begins to "wake up" as the narrative progresses. This former self he calls Phaedrus, after the young sophist in Plato's dialogue of the same name. In Greek, the narrator tells us, Phaedrus means "wolf" (350). Actually, in Greek, Phaedrus means something more akin to "sparkling" (Nussbaum 200), but in the context of the narrative, wolf—accurate or not—forged my own soul connection with this character.

In Phaedrus I finally found an intellectual analogue for my father in the academy. For example, just after Phaedrus has demolished the infamous Chairman of the Committee on Analysis of Ideas and Study of Method (aka: Richard McKeon) in a seminar exchange, Phaedrus walks out of the seminar, and, by extension, out of university life for the last time. As I reread his words, I see my own checkered academic career flash before my eyes:

> Phaedrus the wolf. It fits. . . . Hostility is really his element. It
> really is. Phaedrus the wolf, yes, down from the mountains to
> prey upon the poor innocent citizens of this intellectual commu-
> nity. It fits all right. . . . For him Quality is better seen up at the
> timberline than here obscured by smoky windows and oceans of
> words, and he sees that what he is talking about can never really
> be accepted here because to see it one has to be free from social
> authority and this is an institution of social authority. Quality
> for sheep is what the shepherd says. And if you take a sheep and

put it up at the timberline at night when the wind is roaring, that sheep will be panicked half to death and will call and call until the shepherd comes, or comes the wolf. (386)

Phaedrus the wolf, freed from social authority, pursuing a Zen-like Quality nobody understands, running headlong down a path of psychological self-destruction. Yes, that certainly fits all right.

My own wolf didn't come down the mountain immediately. After his cameo appearance during my PhD orals, he seemed content to lurk in the background, dress in sheep's clothing, mingle with the flock, and obey what the shepherds said. But shepherds aren't stupid; they eventually recognize wolves in their midst. And so in 1974, the same year I read *Zen*, I was denied tenure for the first time just as my first marriage was beginning to unravel. That sheep garb was beginning to pinch.

I didn't think I deserved to be fired, although, come to think of it, few fired people ever do. That's because I was publishing fairly well, teaching very well, and already serving on editorial boards of several prestigious journals. True, I was probably not the consummate "shepherd follower" that my chairperson envisioned (wolves rarely are), but I was just getting started, learning the ropes, getting my feet wet. Surely, I reasoned, that would count for something. When it didn't, I started a precedent I would repeat later. Coming down the mountain as a young hybrid wolf/coyote, I stole into my chairperson's office late one evening. I was there to read my Promotion and Tenure file—sort of a reality check. Much to my surprise, there was one very negative, unexpected letter in my file (another precedent, I might add, that I should have filed away somewhere at the time), but that wasn't what caught my eye. What made my hackles bristle was my own chairperson's icy summary assessment: "Professor Frentz," he wrote, "is abrasive, immature, and lacking in good judgment." In a word, way too wolfish for this mountain. As I crept out of his office that evening, I felt my shape shift just a bit.

I headed home to commiserate with Ben and Amy, with whom I lived at the time. We were all in the same department, and were all riding out the emotional waves of failed relationships. They were, and always will be, my coat from the cold, and that night I really needed one. I had just told Ben and Amy about the letter when Ben started off what would prove to be a rather memorable episode.

"He really said that, in his letter?"

"Yep, right there in black and white."

"What an asshole!" Amy succinctly summed up what we were feeling.

"What's that on your lip?" Ben asked in an apparent non sequitur. "Looks like you've got some zit there or something?"

"Thank you for noticing, but it's just a canker sore," I explained with a trace of irritation. "Got a whole bunch more inside my mouth. Here, wanna see," I added opening up for inspection.

"Oh yechhh!!" Amy blanched. "You *sure* those are canker sores?"

"I'm not sure of much of anything right now. But they're sore and they make me feel cranky. That's pretty good evidence, don't you think?"

"Well, Laura had some of those just last week," she mused. "She thought they were canker sores too, but it turned out she had trench mouth."

"Trench mouth. What's that?" I asked, not really caring if anyone knew.

"I'm not sure what it is, but I do know that it's highly contagious," Amy continued. "So no tongue kissing tonight, you hear? I don't care how god-damned depressed you are, just *deal* with it."

"You absolutely certain that this trench mouth thing is contagious?" I asked, my mind racing right past her and on to darker things.

"Sure is," Ben jumped in, "any form of contact passes it along in a whisper."

"Really?" I added distractedly, a plan now locked in place. "Listen, I know it's late but these damn sores are driving me nuts. I'm gonna run out and get some camphor from an all-night pharmacy, just in case these really are canker sores and not trench mouth. I won't be long."

But I was long—more than two hours. That's because it was not easy to maneuver around campus after midnight. Campus was dangerous at night and always crawling with cops, but I'd been there for five years and knew my way around. I coasted noiselessly into a parking garage just after 2 o'clock. I kept to the shadows until I reached the building that housed our department offices. Silently I slipped inside and dashed to the chairperson's office. There, with wolfish guile, I climbed over his open transom and dropped to the floor. "Now where is the damn thing?" I whispered to myself. "Ah, there she be. Perfect!" All prayers were about to be answered.

It was well after 3 o'clock when I silently slipped into bed. Deep breathing had assured me that Ben and Amy were both fast asleep. Maybe they won't ask, I hoped. At 8 o'clock the next morning we were all sitting around having coffee and saying nothing, the air heavy with anticipation. More coffee, still no questions, but they were both looking at me now with those "Well?" expressions that demanded some sort of response.

"What?" I finally offered when I couldn't stand their beady eyes anymore.

"Guess camphor is tougher to find than you thought, huh?" Amy began, not so subtly.

"So, how far did you have to go before you found it?" Ben pressed.

"I didn't find it. Actually, I didn't even look for it," I confessed.

"So, did you pick someone up?" Ben brightened hopefully.

"No, I went down to school."

"After midnight? You got a death wish?" Amy asked.

"I licked his cup."

"You did *what*?" they asked in unison.

"I licked his fucking tea cup. Left plenty of spit all around the rim. Poetic justice if I give the shitface trench mouth."

Ben took out a pen and began scribbling something on the back of a napkin.

"What now?" I wondered.

"I'm recording this for posterity. You have just committed *the* most heinous social act in the history of academic politics, and I want to note the date, time, place, and circumstances."

"Really? You think it was that good? I just thought it was, well, just some Old Testament justice. So where do you think it would go on my vita?"

"Easy," Amy interrupted. "Under 'Immature, Abrasive, and Lacking in Good Judgment.'"

"No one likes a smartass, Amy," but she was, and I did, although my chair obviously didn't.

History will register that I didn't have trench mouth, and that, aside from a questionable act of oral hygiene, no real harm was done. That would come later. Phaedrus was just waking up; his bite would become worse than his lick.

For those who still don't believe you can step into the same river twice, or that fortune cookies can't tell the truth, a decade later I was fired again. This time, unlike the first, I was married to Janice, and so getting rid of me was, in effect, getting rid of her as well. Becoming wise in the ways of shepherds, I suspected there might have been more to my dismissal than my escalating interludes of howling. So again I decided to check out my Promotion and Tenure file. This time, the political intrigue ran deeper.

Mirroring Pirsig's reconstruction of Phaedrus, I reconstructed—in bits and pieces, through third-hand gossip and veiled innuendo—the scenario that my department, with encouragement from the administration, wanted to hire as chair a highly visible Communication scholar to "turn things around." But, in order to make that happen, the department needed to free up some resources—the administration being far too skeptical of Communication as a legitimate field of study to allocate any new funding. What better way gain the needed resources than to dispose of a wolf and his mate?

I was not happy to have been banished from the mountain again. I was even less happy that Janice, an innocent character in an allegory of which she was unaware, had also been cast aside. Actually, nobody was particularly happy about anything. It was time for a faculty meeting, time for our chair to put the cards on the table, time for some truth telling. But by now I was holding a couple of cards that I was not supposed to have. I knew that the chair had solicited two negative letters for my tenure file. Everyone knew he'd have to address my dismissal, but only I knew that he would have to lie. I just didn't know how he'd go about it.

"I need to apologize to you all," he began humbly.

Pretty decent start, I thought; we all did deserve an apology.

"Obviously, the administration has something in mind for our department other than what we were led to believe," he went on. "As you all know, their promised support has not been forthcoming. I don't know what to make of it, but it is not good news."

Nice grasp of the obvious. Where will he go from here, I wondered.

"I know even less about Tom's case," he lied. "I'm as dumbfounded by his dismissal as the rest of you. Tom has a superb record, is a prolific scholar in rhetorical theory and criticism, garners exemplary teaching evaluations from both students and peers, and has impeccable letters of support."

Actually, I had been hanging in there pretty well until that "impeccable letters of support" line. Then I figured it was time to play my cards, show some teeth, and snarl just a bit. What could he do if I took a chunk or two out of him, fire me? I stood up slowly and turned to face him, feeling a bit like Lon Chaney seeing a full moon in one of his werewolf films. He sensed something was up and braced his back against his chair.

"You lying old pigfucker!" I led off, figuring it was good to begin with honest feelings.

"What did you say?" he stalled.

"I said, 'You lying old pigfucker!'" I repeated with a bit more fervor. "Why don't you tell this faculty how goddamned supportive you've been of me?" I insisted, moving in closer as I did. "Tell them how you inserted two negative letters into my file just to seal the deal."

"I don't know what you're talking about," he lied some more.

"You don't, eh? All right. Let's get my file and open it up—right here, right now. If those two letters aren't there, I'll apologize to the faculty, run twenty laps around campus, moon the chancellor, and kiss your worthless ass. Come on you fossilized old prick," I baited him, "prove me wrong."

He was a beaten old shepherd now and knew there was no way out. He dropped his staff, slumped in his chair, looked down, said nothing, possibly hoping other shepherds would come to his aid. None did. Time for the kill.

"Tell you what. How about I get my file? Then we can all have a look-see together. You up for that?"

"Don't bother," he whispered almost inaudibly. "They're in there."

"Thanks for nothing, asshole. Maybe I can return this little favor some-day," I threatened, but I no longer sounded, or even felt, very threatening. This was not some ruthlessly formidable Richard McKeon, but just a tired, beat-en-down old fart of a chair. I won a badly played skirmish; he won the war. Less than a year later, that highly visible Communication scholar donned the shepherd's garb, dusted off the fallen staff, and began tending his new flock as department chair. The wolf retreated above timberline. But he was loose now, wounded, and hungry for revenge. He wouldn't stay in the high country for long. Colleen would see to that.

Colleen was a graduate student midway through her MA program. I knew of her, had seen her around, and avoided her like the plague. For good reason. The very first time I ever laid eyes on Colleen I hated her, about as thoroughly and intensely as I am capable of hating anyone. This is no great mystery—Colleen was the perfect scapegoat for my shadow. Because I unconsciously feared that I might very well *be* all the things that I so loathed in her, it was much easier to hate her than to face myself. If only I had stayed above timberline, I would not be writing about her here. But I'd caught her scent and was moving in.

Among my other duties that spring, I was director of a mass lecture course entitled, paradoxically enough, "Introduction to Interpersonal Com-munication." I fed my flock with shepherd wisdom once a week, and they baa-baaed it back twice that same week in 25-student discussion sections. As often happens, teaching assistants (lead sheep with bell collars) were handling the discussion sections. Imagine my dismay when, glancing over the list of my TAs for spring, I came across Colleen's name. Given our mutual antipathy, I wondered why, but never asked.

We started off badly right from the get-go. At our first meeting, fourteen TAs and I sat in a circle; Colleen sat alone against the back wall, scowling—my very own black sheep. I carefully reviewed the TA duties: assignments, exams, grading criteria, office hours, deadlines, the usual adminis-trivia. Expecting resistance from Colleen, I went further than usual, offering elaborate, pains-taking reasons for each and every exercise. Colleen bought none of it, just sat there shaking her head. Let's nip this one in the bud.

"Colleen, you seem bothered by all this."

"I just don't see why you need to be involved with our sections," she snapped back, with way more hostility than the situation seemed to demand. "We're perfectly capable of doing this ourselves."

Unfazed, I decided to shift gears, hoping to diffuse her anger within a larger frame.

"Well, some of you are, but some of you aren't, " I continued like the good shepherd, "because some of you are new to this class. But that's not re-ally the point. The point is to have continuity across the sections so that the students will get pretty much the same materials in the same order no matter whose section they are in. Doing the same things at roughly the same times is one way to achieve that continuity."

"*Your* continuity, not mine," she countered.

"No, not really. This continuity was developed over time by the entire fac-ulty," I said, sticking with my larger context strategy. "I'm just implementing it."

"If you say so," she said, but did not mean. With that she got up and walked out.

I know now that I should have stopped her right there, but I was afraid of her. Way too much wolf in this woman. Perhaps even an alpha wolf. But, in terms of the hierarchy, I was the shepherd and she was a sheep, and shepherds aren't supposed to attack their sheep.

This singular exchange was a microcosm of our entire semester together. I'd go over deadlines and duties; Colleen would miss or misunderstand them. I'd schedule TA meetings; Colleen would show up late or not at all. I'd offer sample exam questions; Colleen would critique them, saying that they didn't reflect what she had been teaching. When I tried to trouble-shoot problems between students and TAs, Colleen blamed those problems on the way I was supervising the course.

Things exploded, as these things often do, at final-grade time. Final course grades had to be submitted not later than 72 hours after the final exam for the course in question. At 80 hours, fourteen TAs had their grades in and had departed for the pleasantries of summer. But my grades were still not in because I'd heard nothing from that fifteenth TA.

My chair calls, and I can tell right off he's not a happy camper.

"Where are your grades?"

"Waiting for Colleen," I grumble.

"The Dean's called me twice within the last hour. We can't wait any longer. Why haven't you called her on this?" he asks, with that who's-supervising-this-course-anyway? tone.

So I did what I really didn't want to do. I called Colleen's office.

"Yeah?"

"This is Tom. Can you stop up here for a sec?"

No response. The receiver bangs down, but a couple of minutes later she is standing defiantly in my office doorway.

"The chair just called. The Dean's hassling him for our grades, and that means I need yours. Are you having trouble that I could help with?" This will be my last remark as a shepherd.

"Nothing I can't handle. You'll get them when they're done."

My nostrils flair and my pulse quickens.

"I'm sorry, but that's just not good enough. I need them now. I've had everybody else's since yesterday noon."

"Yeah, well, like I said, you'll get mine when they're ready, and not one minute before!"

Now comes the wolf.

"Look, godammit! I've cut you all of the fucking slack I'm going to. You've stonewalled me ever since the first day of class, and that shit ends right here and now. Get your sorry ass back to your office, crank out those grades, and get them back to me in a nanosecond. You got that, bitch?"

"What did you call me?" she asks incredulously.

"I called you a bitch," I repeat. "No, let me amend that. A fucking bitch!"

"Don't you *ever* call me that!" she shrieks, walking menacingly toward me.

"I *am* calling you that!" I repeat with icy rage. "Now get the *hell* out of my office before I throw you out."

"I don't think you're man enough for the job!"

"Well, we'll just have to see about that, won't we?"

My office was on the third floor of an old fraternity house. Before a wrecking ball destroyed it, paving the way for a new parking lot, the house was a glorious old place with one of those beautiful spiral staircases extending from the lobby all the way to our third-floor offices. I used to lean over that ancient railing, chatting with colleagues and students, listening to the old staircase creak warmly as students made the long climb from the lobby to the offices above.

Now I spin out from behind my desk, grab Colleen by the shoulders, and begin shoving her back toward my door. She knocks my hands aside, pushes me back, and plants her feet, hands firmly set on hips. I charge into her, jamming my left forearm into her mouth, bending her head back, and forcing her out into the hall. She bites down hard and I feel the skin on my arm give way. Her eyes blaze with hate. She struggles against me, but I slowly inch her across the hall and up against the railing. "So long, bitch, you're going down," I whisper hotly in her ear as I slowly bend her over the stairwell railing. Her bite tightens and I now catch flecks of fear in her eyes. I lean in harder. Just a couple more inches and she's gone for good. And then, in an instant, we both tumble over the railing. As we're falling, seemingly suspended in space, her eyes go canine and her mouth changes into a muzzle with razor fangs cutting deeply into my arm. Only now it's less an arm and more a fur-covered foreleg. Downward we spin, seemingly in slow motion, toward the lobby floor—locked in a bestial death spiral.

"Tom! Tom! For God's sake, wake up!"

From someplace far off, I hear Janice's voice and begin coming back.

"Wake up. It's OK. You're here, with me. Everything's all right. You were just having a dream, a nightmare or something."

Unsteadily, I lurch upright in bed, shaking and covered with sweat.

"I killed her," I whisper.

"Killed her? Who? Who did you kill?"

"Colleen."

"Jesus . . . "

"She was a wolf, Babe. I threw her off the balcony near my office, and as we were falling, she changed into a wolf. I think I was a wolf too. We were locked together. We never hit bottom. Just kept falling . . . "

"Listen to me. You didn't kill her. You hear me? *You did not kill her!* You only dreamed it. But stay with the dream, the feelings. They may be crucial. What are you feeling right now?"

I struggle, not sure what I feel, or even if I *can* feel at this moment. Then, almost from a distance, I hear a voice inside me say softly,

"Live by the wolf, die by the wolf."

"What?"

"I'm terrified that if I don't get beyond this wolf thing, I'll either kill through it or be killed by it. I guess that's Colleen's dream gift to me. She and I lived out that reality. I looked into her hateful face and saw my own. It doesn't get much more primal than that."

"No it doesn't, does it? What is it that Jung used to say? Your shadow can be your greatest gift, if you can consciously come to terms with it? Something like that."

Jung probably did say that somewhere. He used to say lots of stuff like that. But it's been hard for me to give up Phaedrus, the wolf. I have so valued what he stands for—principles, strength, courage, Quality. These days, the shepherds have all but eliminated wolves from the academy, always to the detriment of the academy, in my opinion. I keep hoping, with diminishing expectations, that they'll be reintroduced into the hallowed halls someday, as they have been in Yellowstone National Park. But alas, until they are, I cling tightly to a few signs of my old *lupus* persona. I always wear a small wolf necklace that Janice gave me, probably in one of her weaker moments. I still lash out from time to time at old shepherds who abuse young sheep. And, of course, there is this curious mark on my left forearm. It looks like some faded old birthmark, but sometimes, when the light catches it just right, it looks like a scar from a bite. I don't think about it these days. It's just there.

"It's just there." For a long time, I wanted to end this chapter with that. Then I presented an abridged version of this material on an ethnography panel at NCA, and everything changed. Art Bochner was the respondent, and I should have known that he would do more than just cheerlead. He did cheerlead a little—that's Art's gentle nature—but then he got to the hard stuff. "What could it be within the academy," I remember him asking reflectively, "that could produce this sort of rage in you, or in anybody?" Clearly, my actions here were the violent side of the institutional depression that Art had recently addressed. At the time I had no answer, but I remember thinking later, "Professors who remain sheep to the shepherds become depressed, while those who discover that shepherds dominate sheep and kill wolves begin to fight back." That felt right, at least as an intuitive metaphor, if not as a reasoned line of inquiry.

"And I worry," Art continued, turning compassionately toward me, "that you may have done to a student—or, better put, dreamed of doing to a student—what you believe authority figures in the academy have done to you." Ouch! This one really hurt, because Art was so right. Colleen, however nasty or disturbed she might have been, was *not* an authority figure. She was a student, someone I was supposed to shepherd, not smash. But Art didn't know some things, because I didn't tell some things. Colleen was a projection target all right; I told that much. What I didn't tell concerned the specifics of that projection. Although she acted much more like my father than my mother, I felt discounted by Colleen as I had once felt discounted by my parents. Colleen intensified my father's doubts about my manhood and embodied them in a female form. Colleen was not an authority figure in my daily life but, psychically speaking, she sure as hell was, and I now think that I dreamed of doing to her what I so desired, but feared, doing to my parents.

CHAPTER 8

Janice

She's a reason to be reckless, she's the right to rock 'n' roll,
She's exactly what they meant when they told you not to go.
Guy Clark
"Crystelle"

I was beginning to pack up for the day when I heard a gentle tapping at my office door. It was not a raven. I looked up, and my life changed forever. There, in my doorway, I saw a vision that fused the coolest of my mother with the most fevered of my fantasies. A few feet away stood a 5-foot tall, 95-pound platinum blonde with soft brown eyes and a dreamy California tan, wearing a purple mini-dress and sandals. She could have been barefoot, with violets in her hair and grapevines at her feet.

"Hi," she greeted me, but I was still entranced. "I'm Janice Hocker and you're my graduate advisor."

It was my turn to say something but I couldn't make my mouth work.

"Um. . .gosh. . .well. . .Janice. . .what can I do for you?" An infinity of options burst forth in my mind.

"Could you check over these courses and see if they're what I should be taking?"

She moved behind my desk to show me a list she'd jotted down. I tried to focus on the list but her closeness was disorienting and her perfume left me light-headed. Please God, I prayed, don't let spittle drip off my chin.

"You . . . these look fine," I stammered. That was sure to knock her off her feet.

"You new here?" I asked. Why not try again while you're hot?

She ignored my lame patter.

"Yeah, actually I just got in a couple days ago and have been trying to get settled ever since. Otherwise I'd have been by sooner."

I needed a line that didn't sound like a line to set up another meeting with her. What I actually said is as embarrassing now as it was then.

"Well, if anything weird comes up, or if you just need some good restaurants, or if you just need to talk, I'm always here."

"Thanks," she purred, a bit too knowingly, and then was gone just as magically as she had appeared.

I was 33 years old, eclectically educated, fairly well read, recently published, newly married, and doing pretty well at my first academic job. Yet, ten minutes with Janice and I was hopelessly in love. Change was blowin' in the wind.

In Jungian terms, this was a world-class case of *anima* projection (romantic love), in which I invested all of my own feminine sensibilities onto this unsuspecting young woman. Over time, like all romantic lovers, I withdrew those *anima* projections, and when I did Janice transformed from some idealization in my mind into a full-fledged woman on her own. Typically, intimate relationships struggle during these periods. Often they don't survive, particularly when the emerging person cannot quite measure up to the receding ideal. But for me, Janice-the-person is so much deeper, more complex, and emotionally richer than Janice-the-projection that I fell even more deeply in love with the woman than I had with the image. And that's saying something, because the image was pretty damned spectacular in its own right—except, of course, that images have no rights.

Over time it has become obvious that neither Janice-the-image nor Janice-the-woman can save me from my own demons. She cannot rewrite my parental scripts, douse my internal fires, control my emotional outbreaks, or even cure me of cancer. But she can, and does every day, provide the gentle inspiration for me to work on those things myself. She is most certainly a soulmate, if I may be allowed this one fragment from romantic love. As a friend and colleague once told me in regard to Janice, probably not completely in jest, "You're very over-rewarded." So true.

Twenty years into marriage, Janice and I are having breakfast in the sunroom. I have brought coffee on the antique wooden tray Janice's parents gave us several Christmases ago. Mollie, our cat and spiritual child, is asleep on a nearby ottoman with all four paws pointed randomly toward the ceiling in one of her many cute-cat poses. When we first started this Sunday ritual—our relational analogue to church—we got it all wrong. We'd sit there for a few minutes, and then quickly click into to-do lists for the coming week. But, being full professors, it took us only about a month to see this is exactly what we should *not* be doing during this special time. So nowadays we just sit, luxuriate in each other's presence, and see what happens. Today we didn't have to wait long. I was stuck and really needed something to happen.

"Can we talk a bit about my ethnography?"

"Sure."

"Well, yesterday I got back to my cancer stuff," I begin. "I wrote about that frustrating, anger-producing CT scan and how I wanted to deck those two brain-dead nurses. Today I was going to contrast that experience with meeting the throat doc, Kline, and how dependent and respectful I became when he treated me like a person. But when I was getting started, a false note crept in. I came up short and asked, 'What am I trying to do here?'"

"I'm not sure I see the problem," she interrupts.

"Look, " I continue. "I've asked my readers to endure about fifty pages of parental scripts, a veritable zoo of animal personae, and some pretty despicable professional behavior. Now I need to get back to my illness, but what's the tie-in? What am I trying to do here? How is my past related to my present?"

"If you can't bring any wisdom from your past to reconfigure your illness and your present, then what have those first fifty pages been about? Is that it?"

She is with me now.

"Yeah, that's it exactly. All I have so far is, 'I relate to my doctors as I relate to everyone else: If I like 'em, I go belly-up; if I hate 'em, I go into attack mode. That sounds really obvious and inadequate. Sort of I'm-still-where-I've-always-been. You agree?"

"Completely. You've got to say more than that. No, you've got to *do* more than that, for yourself and for your readers. Have you given any thought to where your story will end? You know, if you were writing an academic article, I'd be asking 'What's your thesis?'"

"Well, as you know, the general idea has always been that, since I now have the illness that killed both my parents, I can move beyond the scripts they wrote for me and begin writing and living some of my own. But so far all I seem to be saying is that I write as a sheep and relate, for the most part, as a wolf. While I think that self-characterization is correct, as far as it goes, it hardly seems to qualify as a psychic epiphany that will enable me to live differently from now on."

Janice grows quiet. That usually means she's feeling her way out of my impasse, but needs to choose her words carefully because she knows I'm not going to like what she has to say.

"You're probably not going to like this," she begins tentatively, "but hear me out before you tune out, OK?"

"OK." I stand forewarned.

"I want to revisit our typical division of labor when we write together. I find the literature, do the reading, take the notes, and then we talk about what I've done. Then you sit down, take a deep breath, and type a first draft in four hours. You then drop it in my lap with that little self-satisfied grin on your face, and I agonize over the rewrites for the next three months. Is that fair?" she asks, letting me dangle on the double meaning of "fair."

"That's fair," I admit.

"I don't think you avoid those research tasks because you're lazy or inept—well, you might be inept," she says lightly for my benefit. "No, I think you avoid all those sensing tasks because your creative energies don't flow out of what others have done. What's your classic line here? 'I'm more excited by what I might write than with what others have already written.' I think you avoid most of that front work because it gets in the way of your intuitions, which are the wellspring of your inspiration. Does that still sound right?"

"Of course it does. So what's your point?"

"My point," she leans in hard, "is that you can't craft an innovative way to live with cancer from only memories, dreams, and reflections," her last phrase a reference to Jung's autobiography. "If those resources could do it, you would have already done it and your ethnography would be complete. But now you're stuck, and you can't just drop it in my lap for a quick fix. I think you need to start doing some of those things that I usually do for you."

"Like what?" But I already know what she is going to say.

"Like stop writing for awhile. Do some reading, take a few notes, and see if you can start remembering your dreams again. Get back into your meditation practices. I really believe if your illness harbors a secret for a way to live better the rest of your life, that secret will come to you initially from your unconscious."

"I know you're right, but I want to defend the status quo for a second, OK?" I am blatantly stalling.

"OK, as long as you know that when you say 'I know you're right' it usually means you're not going to do something."

"No, you really *are* right here. But let me tell you why it's so hard for me to let go of my parental tapes. I know you've heard all this, but it's important for me to say it again. The bottom line is that *I like who I am* when I live in relation to those scripts. Although I hide it most of the time because it's not "manly," in certain contexts I like being a sheep. As Hilda taught me, being other-centered and self-sacrificing are wonderful virtues. I also love playing the wolf that I learned from my dad. Of course it's savage, dangerous, and self-destructive, but godammit, it's *manly to a fault*. My wolf is attractive to many people, and it arms me with the charisma that I so value and desire."

"I know that."

Sensing that my defense might work, I push on. "That sheep/wolf opposition is my identity. Students, colleagues, social contacts, even *you* are either attracted to or repelled from me because I embody those two qualities. They make me feel alive. That's why I'm so taken with Pirsig's rebelliousness and Anne Lamott's irreverence. If I erase that opposition, if I—all right, let me say it—if I 'grow up,' I'm afraid I will die psychologically, and perhaps even physically if you factor in my cancer. To be like everyone else is to be dead. I have no desire to be one of Nietzsche's herd. That's what I feel, and that's why it's so hard for me to do anything that might mess with my sheep or wolf. Does this make any sense?" I conclude, sounding a bit more stressed then I intended.

"Of course it makes sense," she says, taking my hand. We sit there for a few moments, allowing her compassion to ease my anxiety. Then she leans in again.

"Let's try another route."

I nod. She closes her eyes, seemingly lost in thought. Then, as much to herself as to me, she says:

"Somehow we need to open some spaces between the mother part of you and the father part, between the sheep and the wolf. I have a feeling that at least part of using your illness to live a better life might be in those spaces."

I had no idea what she was talking about, and she wasn't too sure either, so we just sit there for awhile.

"How do you see yourself when you're at your best?" she asks suddenly.

"That's easy. I like myself best when I empathize with others enough to see things in them that they don't see in themselves. When I have that sort of connection, I create an imaginative context where I can dramatize what I see. This kind of psychodrama is both attractive, because the other plays a major role, and safe, because the person can always disown or dismiss the play if they find their role too uncomfortable."

"Exactly!" she agrees. "That's what *I* love best in you too. But that's not your sheep and that's not your wolf. *That's your trickster!* You *care* for people, *listen* to what they say—whether it's a dream or some life crisis—*invite* them into a wonderfully imaginary world that you create just for them, and then, best of all, you *allow them* to see themselves there as you see them, through playful caricatures of who they've just shown themselves to be. That's pretty special, a high quality way to live."

"My trickster, my trickster," I keep repeating, as if Janice had suddenly reminded me of some long-forgotten mantra. "Of course. The trickster echoes the wolf (through mock attack) and the sheep (through empathy), but moves beyond both into a comic frame that changes the relational structure but does not threaten the faces of the players. Yes, my trickster is still oppositional, still in the me-versus-them mode, but he sees that opposition more as a *necessary tension* to keep hierarchical structures loose and flexible than as an *outright opposition* with the (naïve) intention of breaking those structures down. I can do that. Hell, I've already done that. I don't have to stop writing, start reading, and write down my dreams to remember how," I conclude, with too much defiance and too little deference.

"Fine," she says amicably. "If you ever do stop writing and take up those other things, it's got to come from what you feel, not from what I say. And, who knows? Maybe those new ethnographers are right; since you wrote yourself into this fix, maybe you can write yourself out of it. I don't think so, but it's worth a try."

"That feels right, at least for now. Tomorrow I begin writing myself out of what I've written myself into," I crow, with way too much hubris. "I'll even stick with that CT scan debacle. Perhaps, somewhere in the midst of my relationships with cancer specialists I'll rediscover my trickster. *No problemo.* I can do this."

She smiles that knowing smile.

"Don't look so damned smug, my teen crone. Next Sunday we do *your* psyche."

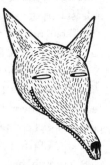

CHAPTER 9

Festum Asinorum

[Jung's dream]. I saw before me the cathedral, the blue sky.
God sits on His golden throne, high above the world—and
from under the throne an enormous turd falls upon the
sparkling new roof, shatters it, and breaks the walls of the
cathedral asunder.

C. G. Jung
Memories, Dreams, Reflections

The receiver is moist in my hand. I feel incredible pressure to ask the right questions and not forget the answers.

"What sort of tests?" I begin sheepishly, and that *is* the right question for now.

"I want to start with a CT scan of your pelvic area," Dr. Logan reasons, "because that's the most likely place we'll find the primary, and, if this thing's spread anywhere other than to your lymph nodes, we'll most likely find evidence of that in the pelvic region too."

"Why not an MRI?" I ask, because I've had MRIs before and know what they entail, and because I want to sound reasonably knowledgeable about medical technology.

"Because MRIs don't imprint clearly areas with moving parts—like lungs, bowels, bladders, or hearts. We do CT scans for those things," comes his response.

"Then what?" I push, wanting to know as much about what may be ahead of me as is possible.

"Let's just see what we find with the CT scan, OK?" he dodges, apparently deciding that he doesn't have enough data right now to predict my future.

I try not to think about cancer growing inside me, but I can't not think about it. I think about it all the time—endlessly—fear and dread now replacing the sense of "destiny" that came first. I want all the tests now, today, within the hour, sooner! But the medical profession doesn't work that way. There are hundreds, thousands, of equally anxious people all wanting to find out their fate yesterday. Thank God I live in a small town. My CT scan is scheduled for the following Monday.

It is nearly 5 o'clock and already I don't like the feel of this. I'm in a mid-sized regional hospital, our town's best approximation of a medical bureaucracy. My appointment was scheduled for 45 minutes ago. Janice, a mutual friend Paula, and I sit in the typical waiting area. Fake wooden tables, two-year-old magazines, bored attendants behind a desk, and anxious patients, most accompanied by equally anxious families, going into and coming out of the CT scan room. By 5:20 we're the only three left. As I head up to the desk, I catch a sideways glance from Janice that pleads "Be nice!" The young woman behind the desk has her back to me and is talking to another attendant. I wait patiently, being extremely nice. The second attendant sees me, but says nothing.

"Excuse me?" the niceness now straining ever so slightly.

"Yes?" the attendant turns around, looking surprised and slightly irritated.

"I'm Tom Frentz and I had a 4 o'clock appointment for a CT scan," I offer, looking pointedly at the wall clock behind her desk.

She glances down at her schedule.

"Oh yeah. Well, they're running a bit behind this afternoon. Have you drunk any dye yet?"

"No, am I supposed to?"

"Yeah. Just a sec."

She gets up, heads over to a small refrigerator, takes out a plastic bottle, and, handing it to me, says, "Here, drink this and they'll be right with you."

I gag down a pinkish-white slime that tastes like sour cream laced with Drano. I slink back to my seat and begin reading a *Sports Illustrated* article for the third time. It's either that or *Southern Living*, and I've had about all of that I can take for one afternoon.

At 6:24 two tired-looking medical technicians stick their heads through the waiting room door.

"Mr. France?" one asks.

"That would be me."

"Follow me."

I follow them into a large room that houses what looks like a partially completed MRI unit in the center—the CT scan contraption. The two women are studies in contrast. One is tall and thin. Earlier, her make-up was probably where she wanted it, but now it's spread out a bit, giving her an indistinct, ghostly cast. The other is short, stocky, nondescript and never seems to notice that I'm even in the room. She just heads off into some "control room" where, I presume, she'll monitor whatever the CT scan registers on the computer screens.

"Just leave your clothes on the chair," says the tall one, whose expression is meant to be a smile, but really isn't. No feelings here. Just some well-rehearsed lines with facial accompaniments that are, like Richard Nixon's once were, a microsecond late. I turn my back to them, shed my clothes, climb into the all-purpose, backside-beware hospital gown, and lie down resignedly on the CT scan gurney. Still not looking at me, the tall technician begins fussing with something next to me.

"Ever had one of these, Mr. France?" she asks, still without looking or caring.

"Nope. Don't believe I've had the pleasure," I drone back, trying to model back her measured indifference. "But I've had a few MRIs and . . . "

"It's no big deal really," she interrupts without listening. "We'll just start an IV and then . . . "

"Excuse me," I interrupt, not indifferent anymore, "I didn't think CT scans were invasive. You see, while trying to find something to do for the last three-and-a-half hours in the waiting room, I had the chance to read, more carefully than you might imagine, the literature on CT scan procedures, and there's no mention of an IV."

"Yeah, well, sometimes they're not used, but in order to see any tumor or obstruction in your system, we need to inject a contrasting dye as we take the pictures. This only takes a sec. and then . . . "

She's going way too fast. I'm not paranoid about needles and IVs, but, like most everyone, they're not my favorite recreational drugs. I put on my best let's-get-this-right-the-first-time expression, but she's still not looking. She misses the vein by a country mile.

"Damn. Silly vein of yours keeps moving," she says, blaming my vein for her ineptness. She jams the needle harder the second time. Might makes right.

"Goddamn! That sure felt great! You ever done this before?"

No response.

"Now just lie back and . . . "

"Excuse me, but I *am* lying back," I inject sort of obviously.

" . . . and when I tell you, raise your arms over your head, OK?"

"Gee, I'd really love to, you see, but I've got this IV thing in my arm. Remember?"

"Oh don't worry, Mr. France. There's plenty of line for you to raise your arms."

"I'm just a visitor here, of course, but it sure doesn't look like there's plenty of line," I worry.

She's still not listening, but rather heading off to the control room to join her partner in crime.

"Can you hear me, Mr. France?" someone asks from the control room.

"Loud and clear."

"All right then, we're going to move you under the CT scan now. Put your arms over your head."

As I raise my arms, I watch the thin tube from my IV tighten as the gurney moves back. Tighter, tighter, no more slack now, but the gurney is still moving. I feel a sharp pain as the IV pulls out of my arm and drops to the floor.

"I'm usually not one to say 'I told you so,'" I begin, "but the IV's now on the floor and my arm seems to be bleeding a little."

Movement in the control room. The tall technician re-emerges and walks sullenly toward me, looking slightly pissed off. She snaps the IV up off the floor, tosses it into a trash bin, grabs a fresh one from a drawer, and heads over to me.

"Guess we didn't allow for your arms and the movement of the platform," she complains in what is about as close to an apology as I'm likely to get.

I cut her no slack. Somebody is paying way too much for this sort of indifference.

"Do you suppose that 'we' might allow for both of those things this time? I can't speak for you here, but I'm just not having fun anymore," the wolf says, barely in check.

No response. We all just want this to be over now. She hooks another IV in my other arm, adds enough leader line to stretch to the next county, cranks me back under the machine, and, for the next fifteen minutes or so, photographs me from the outside in.

"Sorry about that IV, Mr. France." I don't really think she is.

"Yeah, I am too."

I collect my clothes and some of my composure, they collect whatever it is they collect, and we go our separate ways. It's now after 7 o'clock. As Paula, Janice, and I make our way out of this planet of the apes, I try to stay with my feelings. I'm sorry it got so late. I'm sorry the technicians were tired. I'm sorry they couldn't relate. I'm sorry they don't give a damn about what they do. I'm sorry that I have cancer, wherever it is, and they don't seem to care much about that either. But mostly, I'm sorry I couldn't craft a tricksterish way to combat their clicked-off sourness. If this episode is any indication, recovering my trickster is going to be a lot harder than I figured.

Three days later I'm back in Dr. Logan's office. Aside from his unusual first name, Gareth is pretty usual. He's stockily built with a subtle gracefulness that doesn't seem to match his overall presence. He has a round face, deep-set eyes, and wears tear-shaped glasses. He always wears the TV doctor uniform, a starched, white, mid-calf coat. He carries a pen in his right hand even when he shakes my hand, sort of like Bob Dole. Perhaps it's to keep people from damaging his most vital surgical instrument. I liked Gareth immediately, but I'm not sure everybody does. There's something enigmatic about him, something that many might see as aloofness, but I don't. I'm there for the results of the CT scan.

"Well, what's the deal?" I ask, not sure that I really want to know.

"Clean as a whistle."

"What do you mean, clean as a whistle?"

"I mean there's no sign of a primary anywhere. Nothing in the pelvic region, which is what I expected. Nothing in the lungs. Lymph nodes under your arms as normal as apple pie. Very strange."

"This is good, right? I mean if I don't have a primary tumor somewhere, then all I have is this lymph node shit, and you whacked those out." I'm feeling better already.

"Well, it's a little more complicated than that." He says this slowly, trying not to deflate my newfound confidence without misleading me.

"If we can't find a primary tumor," he continues, "that means an unspecified malignancy is moving through your bloodstream and we don't know where it is or how to treat it. This condition is known as UPS. It's very rare. I've never seen it before."

"UPS? Gareth, that's a goddamned mail service!" I say, going for a very unfelt trickster moment.

"In cancer terms it's 'unidentified primary syndrome,' and it's not a very positive diagnosis. When it occurs—and again, that's not very often—it's classified as type IV cancer, where type I is the best and there is no type V."

I'm stunned and scared. What sounded like very good news was now sounding very bad.

"So now what?"

"Well, now I think we should . . . "

He stops in mid-sentence and peers at one part of the scan.

"Wait. Here's something."

"Something bad?" I ask, sliding around next to him to see.

"Here, at the base of your throat. See that hazy dot? That's a tiny, dark mass. Now I really don't think it's the primary, " he cautions, "because if your groin cancer had originated in your throat, your lungs would have been invaded on its way down, and your lungs are fine. But let's let Randy Kline check this out just to be sure."

"Who's Randy Kline?"

"A good friend and one of the better throat doctors in town. Knowing Randy, he'll see you real soon."

"Soon is good."

Janice and I are in Randall Kline's waiting room the very next day. This is a different place with a different feel. It's not exactly *Marcus Welby MD*, but it's definitely not one of those hi-tech shops either. It's pleasantly run-down, with chairs and tables showing signs of too many infant kicks. The aged magazines have no covers—mystery reads, all. The staff seems almost happy to be there. We don't wait long. In Randall's small office, Janice and I hold hands, hoping for something. Almost immediately, the door opens and a gentle, focused man walks in.

"Dr. Frentz?"

"Randall?"

"Yes."

He takes a second, looks at me carefully, then over at Janice, then back to me.

"This is pretty scary, isn't it?" he asks as if he really knows.

My stomach churns, Janice looks away, and he softens still more.

"Look," he says quietly, "I'm almost certain that we're not going to find anything in your throat, but I want to make sure because Gareth wants to make sure. And then," he adds warmly as if knowing what we need to hear most, "I want to help you anticipate a bit more clearly what's ahead of you."

As he passes me in search of a tongue depressor, he lays his hand reassuringly on my shoulder. Not many men, except maybe Bill Clinton, can touch other men they've just met in that way without it feeling all smarmy and invasive.

"All right now, here's what I'm going to do. Your CT scan showed this slight mass right behind your left tonsil. In order for me to see that area, I'm going to have to depress your tongue pretty far down. And that means that you're going to gag—you won't be able to help it, just an automatic reflex. So just gag, I'll get in and out quick as a flash, OK?"

"OK," I say, and then add, "Should Janice leave?"

"Nah," Randall chuckles, "you'll gag just fine with her here."

With great care, he presses my tongue down, I gag, he swabs something way back in there, and then it's over.

"Well, you don't have cancer in your throat. That mass is just a common tonsil shadow that CT scans pick up sometimes. I figured that all along, Gareth probably did too, but now we know for sure."

"So now what?" I ask, not knowing whether to be relieved or concerned. "Gareth says that an unidentified primary syndrome is bad news," I add, hoping that Randall will tell me that Gareth is wrong.

"He's right, but it's a tricky deal. Sometimes a cancer spreads, as yours apparently has, and then the body's natural immune system kills off the primary source of the spreading. That's often why we can't find it. In those cases, what matters most is what sort of cancer we're dealing with and how far it's spread. In your case, squamous cell carcinoma is typically a very slow growing cancer and yours seems well contained in two lymph nodes in your pelvic region. So, even if we can't find a primary source, this may not be quite as grim as you've been led to believe. I'm not peddling false hope here," he assures us, "I'm just trying to expand the context for your fears."

Here's a specialist, a throat guy, with no previous contact with me, called in, in all likelihood, as a favor to Gareth, who's relating to Janice and me as if we were the two most important people in the world. It's a rare moment in modern medicine and I imprint it well. Even as it's unfolding, I sense that it won't happen again, at least not quite like this. I have just met one of the rare good shepherds in the medical profession. It's an honor to be a sheep in his presence, even if my life now, not just my manhood, is at stake.

So right here, in the earliest stages of my cancer odyssey, I felt constricted to only two choices: baa like a sheep or howl like a wolf. With the scan technicians, my sheep-like dependency on their "expertise" quickly gave way to some much-deserved wolfishness. By contrast, with Gareth Logan, and more completely with Randall Cline, I hunkered down in sheep mode, tolerating it with Gareth, and actually enjoying it with Randall. But neither sheep nor wolf is appropriate here, because both beasts tacitly legitimate what medical specialists already do far too well already: use the rigid structure of the medical community to objectify me and see my body as an ensemble of parts. Eventually, treating my body as parts will kill all my animal personae. As I quickly discovered, this implicit organizational structure is endlessly replicated through the ordinary everyday chitchat between doctors and patients.

I remembered how stunned Arthur Frank was when an ultrasound specialist said of a large mass discovered behind Frank's groin, "This will have to be investigated" (50–51). The trick, as Frank learned well, was to resist this kind of talk and the relational disconnects that it fosters without simultaneously resisting the important care medical specialists have to give. Whatever this trick was, it was going to take a lot more than my parents had given me.

Frank resisted by enacting subtle, culturally shared norms of human recognition that forced medical people to see him as an ill person, not as a diseased object. Thus, when an obviously uncomfortable anesthesiologist tried to explain what he would be doing during Frank's next-day surgery without ever looking at him, Frank retaliated with:

> When he was leaving, I did the worst thing to him that I could
> think of: I made him shake hands. A hand held out to be shaken
> cannot be refused without direct insult, but to shake a hand is to
> acknowledge the other as equal. The anesthesiologist trembled
> visibly as he brushed his hand over mine, and I allowed myself to
> enjoy his discomfort. (55)

But I'm not Arthur Frank and sophisticated subtleties have never been my long suit. So, whereas my own tendency in his particular situation would have been to say something dysfunctionally wolfish like "Look pod person. You overmedicate me, I underpay you." I know that's not the answer here either.

Neither wolf nor sheep, Janice keeps saying. But what else is there? My trickster, of course, but how can I access him with medical people? So one day, when I'd reached my confusion quota for the day, I just gave up and went for a long walk. On my way back, from out of nowhere, the name "Larry" popped up. The only Larry I know around here is my GP of 15 years, Larry Crandall. As I thought about Larry, I recalled a rather memorable conversation we had that led, although in a rather circuitous route, to the discovery of cancer. Now *that* sounded way too synchronistic to ignore. Perhaps, just perhaps, one of those elusive trickster moments is lurking back there in what we said to one another.

I was referred to Larry in 1985 when I first moved here, and he's been my doctor ever since. We've both aged some since then. These days he sports short-cropped gray hair and has a slight middle-aged paunch. Larry has a busy, expressive mouth, and playful gray eyes, and he always wears the same thing: a faded, button-down jeans shirt, khaki pants, and a pair of godawful shoes that squeak when he walks. We hit it off immediately. Whatever the malady, our routine now unfolds something like this: I wait in his tiny office, he opens the door reading my chart and says, without looking up, "Tom, how you doing?" I say, "Not worth a shit or I wouldn't be here." He grins, looks up, we shakes hands, and then he goes off on the topic of managed health care for about ten minutes. When he stops to take a breath, I jump in and go off about whatever's ailing me. Then we both go off from there.

Today, in early January 2000, starts out pretty ordinary.

"I've had some bleeding from my rear," I begin. "It's probably just those hemorrhoids you noticed before, but I guess you should check it out."

"You know the routine," he agrees, fumbling in a drawer for the hated sigmoidoscope.

"Assume the position," he commands, doing his best Marquis de Sade.

"Geez, Larry. Can't you just take a nice x-ray or something?"

"Look, you're the one with the bad butt."

"Yeah, but . . . "

"No buts, just give me yours."

"Easy for you to say."

"All right, my man. Here comes the worst three minutes of your day. Roto-rooter," he sings. "Hold it. There . . . OK . . . we're in. You doing OK?"

"Oh, great! Why don't you just check my tonsils as long as you're up there that far?"

"Don't tempt me."

"I always tempt you. That's why I'm not like your other patients."

"Shut up now, goddamnit. Let me look around. This isn't easy, you know."

"Yeah? You should feel it from my end."

And then, with about 15 feet of plastic tubing up my ass, inspiration strikes.

"Larrrr-yyyy?" This in my best imitation of how baseball fans used to pimp Daryl Strawberry by yelling "Darrrr-yyyyllll."

"What now?"

"How long have we known each other?"

"How the hell should I know? Ten, maybe fifteen years. Why?"

"Well . . . I was just wondering . . . I'm having feelings that I can't explain."

"You hurt up here somewhere?"

"No, no, they're not those kind of feelings, Larry. They're not physical. Well . . . I guess they are, sort of. They're more, well, more . . . Geez, this is really hard!"

I'm cruising now and he has no idea what's coming.

"All right, I'm just going to come right out with it. Larry, when we're this close, do you have any feelings for me as a person?"

He tries hard not to laugh, which I appreciate because of where his space probe is just now.

"None whatsoever!" he finally spits out. "You're a patient, for crissake, patients aren't persons. I thought you knew that." Then quickly, "Now don't distract me or I'll charge you extra for helping."

I will not be deterred.

"You know you're hurting me, right?"

"Right! Now be a brave little professor and shut up!"

"God I love it when you talk nasty to me."

"All right, that's it," he says. "You're just so full of shit. Did you know that?"

Now it's my turn to laugh.

What I see here is that when I act out of my trickster role, I destroy the structure but not the person. This is, I think, a very important rhetorical strategy: Savage the structure (a dash of wolf), but save the face (a pinch of sheep). Obviously, for this trickster frame to be established, Larry had to play along. But when he did, we were able to enter a comic world of the trickster, and to relate more personally without ever compromising his professionalism.

This conversation did more than create a trickster-inspired space for my doctors and me. It also began my medical experience with cancer. For, when the sigmoidoscopy proved inconclusive, Larry referred me to Gareth for the turbocharged version known as a colonoscopy. Although that test didn't find anything either, just before the colonoscopy I discovered the two swollen lymph nodes whose subsequent removal revealed the cancer.

I now had one small space and one large illness. What I didn't have was the location of that elusive primary. Larry didn't know, Randall didn't know, and Gareth didn't know. One CT scan and two MRIs didn't reveal anything. But I was rediscovering my trickster, and, as such, I now I had a hunch. I was back in Gareth's office, and he was not a happy camper.

"I'm stumped. We've probed, prodded, and photographed every inch of you and there's just no sign of any primary. I'm afraid we're going to have to stick with that UPS diagnosis," he sighs, "and go from there."

But I'm not ready to go from there.

"It's in my ass, Gareth," I say, with absolute certainty but no data.

"What did you say?" he asks, without really connecting.

"I said, 'It's in my ass!' and it is. Look, this is my destiny. Lots of people already think I'm an asshole. I've bared it to moon the best and brightest in my field from time to time. Trust me on this one, Gareth. Is there anything you can do that you haven't already done?"

He thinks about this for a minute.

"Well, I suppose I could take some blind biopsies, but they're usually pretty inconclusive. To be honest, usually they're just a waste of time."

"They won't be this time. Trust me," I add confidently.

Since he doesn't have any better idea, a week later he biopsies all four quadrants of my beleaguered butt. Two days later he calls with the pathology report, sounding almost incredulous. "Well I'll be goddamned. You were right. Two of the four tissue samples reveal small traces of squamous cell carcinoma *in situ*. So the bad news is, we've found more cancer, but the good news is that we've finally found that elusive primary, and that's going to make things a helluva lot easier. Now it's your turn to trust me."

The treatment protocol for anal cancer with lymph node involvement is pretty straightforward. Twenty-five radiation treatments to the pelvic area coupled with two 96-hour injections of chemotherapy, one during the first week of treatment, the other during the last. Five weeks. I can do that. My mother did that, only for much longer. My father did that, for about the same time. Of course, they're both dead. Best not to go there. Just buckle up, swill some hooch, bite down, and have at it. Double trouble for my ass—nuke it from without and poison it from within. That should do it. I sure hope that will do it.

It is early April and I'm at the central radiation center in an adjacent suburb to get "simulated," not in any postmodern sense, but in the distinctly modernist medical sense of marking where the radiation should be directed. I call this event "targeting" because it's where somebody paints a bulls-eye that the radiation technologists try to hit. Since misses aren't allowed, I'm already wondering whether there'll be some dummy practice sessions with rubber bullets.

I look around. Not bad as waiting rooms go. High, beamed ceilings in taupe. Claret-colored, upholstered chairs with *faux* oak arms. Gray and white swirl carpet. The whole motif reeks of early Ralph Lauren *sans* the polo guy. I'm a little uptight. Save for my non-contact with my mom and dad years ago, this is my first prolonged experience with a facility geared toward cancer patients. I look around again, noticing the people this time. I count ten waiting with me. A woman sits across from me, head down, eyes closed, obviously not having a good day. Behind me I can hear "Good Morning, America." For most of us here, this isn't. Then I notice a pattern. It turns out that those who "look healthy" are, in fact, healthy. They turn out to be family and friends waiting for those who are not so healthy and who, in all likelihood, are getting their radiation breakfasts in another part of the facility.

A medical staff person emerges from behind closed doors and says "Mr. France?" "Close enough." I follow her through the doors and down a hall. We stop about halfway and she says "You can change in here." "In here" is an open room with lockers. "Just remove your trousers and put the gown and robe on. Leave the gown opening in front, and lock your stuff in here," she continues handing me key number 33. Ron Dayne's number when he played football at Wisconsin. I guess I'm looking for a good luck sign wherever I can find it. I emerge looking sick. Everybody here wearing a gown and robe looks sick, that's how you know. All the chairs are taken, and so I sit on a scale. But not for long. A nurse approaches with a guy in tow.

"Are you waiting for treatment?" she asks cheerily.

"Yep."

"Well, I wonder if I could borrow your 'seat' to weigh this gentleman?" she asks hesitantly.

"Sure, but you don't need to. He weighs 163 pounds." I say pulling this number out of my ass, which, lest we forget, is where the cancer is.

He sits, I stand, she gasps.

"My God! He *does* weigh 163 pounds—on the nose."

"What? You thought I'd lie to you? In here? Geez! And you'd better treat me right, because I know how much you weigh too."

Here it is again. Another trickster space. Some authoritative structure compromised, a bit of intuitive luck, and all faces preserved. I think I'm getting the hang of this.

I am getting resettled in a grotesque fake leather La-Z-Boy when I hear "Hi! You Mr. France?"

"Close enough."

"I'm Cameron and I'll be doing your simulation today," he announces. "Follow me, please."

Cameron's about my height, heavy set, with a short buzz cut. He's decked out in traditional radiation tech garb: white lab coat, rumpled jeans, and Nike running shoes. We walk down a long, wide hall and enter a room with SIMULATION emblazoned above the door.

"You ever had a CT scan?" he asks, fumbling with some gadgets on the scanner.

"Yeah, it sucked bad."

"Really? That's odd. They're usually no big deal."

"Maybe not, but they become more of a big deal when an IV's involved."

"Ah, you had the Technicolor one. Yeah, they're a bit more of a problem. But none of that today. No IV, no dye, just some pictures."

I relax noticeably.

"When I fire this thing up," he cautions, "it's gonna sound like gravel rattling inside an empty beer can. Marvels of modern medicine. I'll be imaging you for only about ten minutes," he explains, "but you'll be lying here for another fifteen. I'm not out for coffee or anything, just studying the data and figuring out where to mark you."

"How do you mark me?"

"With felt-tipped pens—the general target area in black, the bull's-eye in red. Then I'll cover the marks with transparent strapping tape so you can't wash them off in the shower."

"What if you get the marks in the wrong place?" I worry.

This one brings Cameron up short. He pauses, thinks about it a second, and then a wicked smile slowly spreads across his broad face.

"Well, in that case, I guess we'd accidentally sterilize you." He pauses to let this one register. Then, "Would that be a problem?"

I guess I'm not the only trickster working here. The markings go on without a hitch or an erasure. On my way out, I see the weigh-in nurse. "One thirty-three," I whisper as I pass, purposely guessing low, and she beams.

Here was another space, tiny, to be sure, but very important. In some of these interactions, I made others feel good about themselves by combining empathy and humor in a way that enhanced rather than diminished who I am. I like that.

Six days later I show up for my first treatment. I sign endless forms. The last one summarizes the costs for twenty-five radiation treatments: $10,987. That's roughly $440 a pop, and since a pop lasts only 7 seconds, it's approximately $63 a second. The receptionist points me towards another small room with lockers. "You can change in there. Wear the same gown all week. On Friday, put it in that bin over there and we'll have you a fresh one on Monday. You can leave your socks on if you like." I change, leave my socks on, sit in the small waiting room, and leaf idly through *Modern Maturity*.

Just as I turn a page, in walks Heather. Be still, my heart. Cameron told me that someone named Heather would, in all likelihood, supervise my treatments, but he didn't prepare me for the woman behind the name. Heather must be about 5' 10" with an oval face, perfect complexion, huge ice-blue eyes, a mane of jet black hair cascading down her back, and an overbite to die for. She just stands there smiling; I just sit there staring. I already know that I'm not being modernly mature. It's not so much her drop-dead physical beauty that melts me (well, it's partly that) as it is a twinkling mischievousness in her eyes. She's got to know the effect she has on men—especially men in here, who, like me, undoubtedly feel vulnerable, frightened, and not all that manly. If ever there was a set-up for me to kick into those old mother tapes, this was it.

"Hi Tom, I'm Heather."

"Hi Heather, I'm Tom."

"I know," Heather says, forgivingly. "Well, you ready to do this thing?"

"I guess."

She smiles, turns, and heads off down a hall toward the radiation room with me in tow. As we walk, Heather chirps about the procedure.

"OK. Here's the deal," she begins. "When we get in there, you lie down on the padded gurney. I'll put an alloy mold over your pelvic area that will keep the radiation directed to where we want it to go. Then I'll place a flat piece of goofy plastic—you know, the same stuff they make those slimy bugs out of that they sell at Wal-Mart—over the area where you had the lymph nodes removed. The plastic will intensify the radiation in that area, just in case Dr. Logan missed a few cells."

She pauses here, probably to let this sink in, or to see if I have any questions, or just to make sure that I've not turned and fled. Since I'm still there, she starts up again.

"After we get the mold and plastic in place, I'll head out to a control room and you'll be on your own. Don't worry," she anticipates, "I'll talk to you the whole time over an intercom. I'll be aligning the radiation 'gun' with the computerized images of you that were marked during simulation. When I get you in my cross hairs, I'll ask you to lie still, and I'll shoot you for approximately 7 seconds from overhead. Then I'll come back in, remove all the junk, rotate the machine underneath you, and then give you another 7 seconds from behind. Whole operation will take about 5 minutes. Got it?"

"Got it," I say, a helluva lot more confidently than I feel.

I hold onto it until I get to the room itself. Then I start to lose it. "Danger! Radiation!" in huge block red letters looms ominously over the door. The door itself is twelve inches of solid lead hung on hinges that could support the *Titanic*. I flash back on those horrific Hiroshima pictures. Then I remember my mother's charcoaled chest. I'm pretty stressed out, but I don't want Heather see that, although I'm sure she does.

I enter the room and lie down stiffly on the gurney. Initially, it feels just like any other gurney. But then, without warning, it feels *real* different. Heather breezily flips up my already-revealing gown, blithely tucks my pre-shrunk manhood out of sight between my legs, and begins to position the goofy goo on my groin. What's the line from "Hotel California"? "This could be heaven or this could be hell." In that single, omigod instant, Heather opened another space; now there was no way I could relate to her as I once did to my mother. I wasn't about to miss this trickster moment.

"Heeaa-therrr?" I purr, reprising the intonation once used with Larry.

"Yee-eesss?" she purrs back.

"Could you please do me a *big* favor?"

"And what might that be?"

"Could you please not nuke 'Mr. Happy'?"

Heather tosses her mane back and lets go a big Julia Roberts laugh. We both just let the moment hang there.

"Not to worry. 'Mr. Happy' is in no danger from me."

I breathe a mock sigh of relief. As she heads out, Heather pauses, turns, and shoots me a wicked wink.

"You ready?" I hear her say over the intercom.

"Fire at will," I answer back heroically.

"Think I'll fire at Mr. Happy. Oops! Sorry. Think I'll fire at Dr. Tom, OK?"

"OK, just don't miss."

She's right about the time too. When I hear the radiation buzz begin, I count "1-one-thousand, 2-one-thousand . . . " and somewhere between 6-one-thousand and 7-one-thousand, the buzzing stops. Heather bounces back, carefully removes the heavy mold, peels back the goo, and then starts giggling again. She's doing *something* to my stomach. I'm thinking, probably some part of the procedure she forgot to mention. I should have known better.

"There!" she says triumphantly. "Something to remember me by."

I sit up and look down at my belly. There, over my navel, she has drawn a face with the navel as its mouth.

"Will this come off?"

"Not a chance."

"But what will I tell Janice?"

"I'm not really sure, but you'd better come up with something good. If she doesn't kill you, I'll see you tomorrow. Y'all take good care of 'Mr. Happy' now, y'hear?"

With that, she helps me up, and heads me out. Although radiation, I would come to discover, has a cumulative effect that goes from nothing to bad to worse, Heather has a cumulative effect too that goes from good to better to best. Our banter in this world was extremely important because I could relate to Heather as a woman without ever losing touch with myself as a man. Equally important, I could do this without ever compromising her skills as a medical professional who was trying to save my life.

Neither Cameron nor Heather was a medical authority figure to me. It is one thing to carve out little trickster spaces with people not too high up on the medical food chain, but quite another to pull that off with a bona fide heavyweight. The weightiest of heavies goes to my oncologist, Thaddeus J. Carlson.

As soon as the pathology report on my lymph nodes came back, my close friend Paula, who is extremely well connected in the local medical community, began mulling over the available oncologists. Her recommendation surprised me.

"You know," she said one evening, "most of the university people work with Malcolm Woodward. He's Ivy League, has a quick, sarcastic wit, like you, and most say he's a genius. But, the more I think about it, the more I think you should go with Thad Carlson. He's—I don't know—I just feel you'd connect better with Thad than you might with Malcolm."

"Sounds good to me," I say, having no reason to doubt Paula. "Besides, my ex-wife's father was named Malcolm."

"Well then, that just cinches it, doesn't it?"

Janice and I meet Thad for the first time in early March. We're both terrified because we've not located a primary cancer yet, and because we know that when you have to see an oncologist, it's not exactly a good sign. He walks in, shakes hands warmly, and sits down. I'm struggling to pin down a first impression. He's very hard to read. I like his eyes immediately—dark brown, concerned, caring, but complex. He looks right at me, another plus. No hospital getup for him, but a costume nevertheless. He wears a white button-down, 100% cotton, oxford-cloth shirt, no jacket, khaki slacks, oxblood Rockports, and a hand-tied bow tie. Paul Simon, the democratic senator from Illinois, is the last guy I remember who wore one of those. Well, actually, my dad did too.

As Thad studies my chart, I study his name. Thaddeus (I'm thinking prissy) relates to old money . . . begot from conservative stock . . . sounds Yankee . . . so what's he doing down south? Back to the eyes. Do I catch hidden mirth in there somewhere, or do I just need to relieve some tension? The more I look, the more I see. It's not as up-front and in your face as with Heather, but it's there. I'm absolutely sure of it. I know I can get Thad to play with me, but I'm not sure how. There's no chance this first go-around. Thad affirms what both Gareth and Randall already have told me, that a UPS diagnosis isn't good. Mainly, we just get acquainted and make another appointment to review test results.

Several weeks later, after the biopsies revealed where the primary is, we meet again. I don't think he's even changed clothes—same white shirt, same khaki slacks, same Rockports, same—no, different—bow tie. This time he's definitely more upbeat.

"Hell, I can cure this," he says with an air of confidence I'm thrilled to hear. Words to live by, literally.

"Really?" Janice and I say, in unison.

"Yep, wanna see the stats?"

We do, so he slips out and comes back carrying a huge black book.

"Let's see. Anal . . . anal . . . anal cancer," he muses as he flips through pages. "Ummm . . . OK, here we are, page 1328. In Finland—yep, here we go—nine cases of anal cancer with lymph node involvement. With radiation and chemotherapy, the cure rate is over 70 percent. It drops to just over 35 percent with radiation alone, and lower than that if more than three lymph nodes are involved." Sensing, perhaps, that as these survival rates drop, my confidence level might be dropping too, he quickly adds, "But all of these cases involved tumors in the anal canal and you don't have a tumor. Your cancer is *in situ*, meaning that it hasn't penetrated the surface tissues. So I would say that your odds are even better than those in this study," he concludes.

"That's a damn small sample," I say skeptically, forgetting for a moment that I am a recovering social scientist.

"Well, squamous cell anal cancer with lymph node involvement is a pretty rare statistical event. Yours is the first case I've ever seen and I've been at this for awhile."

"So what's next?" I ask hopefully.

"Why don't you two think over what you want to do. There's no immediate urgency, although I wouldn't dally around forever. If you want to go for the radiation/chemotherapy combination, and I'd strongly recommend that, the protocol's pretty straightforward, and we'll get you set up."

This is a no-brainer. I get a second opinion on the lymph node biopsies from M. D. Anderson, the huge cancer research center in Houston, but once the diagnosis is confirmed Janice and I order the combination platter. Soon after Cameron simulates me for radiation, I head back to see Thad about chemotherapy. Third meeting, same costume. I'm thinking, this is a game, right? I say the right words, he peals off the Clark Kent garb, and poof, right there before my eyes, Superoncologist! Although I'm feeling much more confident about my future, I'm really apprehensive about chemotherapy. I can replay way too many bad parental tapes here. I need another space, but Thad's provided none so far.

While he's looking at my chart, I'm looking for an opening.

"What's your schedule like next week?"

"Fine, why?"

"I need to see you in my other office to install a catheter."

Whoa, my stomach turns upside down. If this is oncology's version of simulation, I'm thinking, it's already not half simulated enough for me. Then, a mini-inspiration hits.

"Thad. I don't want you to stick anything up my pee-pee. My cancer's in my ass, not my dick, remember?" Well, I figure I might as well try something.

Nonplused, he goes for the big yawn response.

"It's no big deal, really. A catheter's just a thin, flexible tube that I run into a vein just under your collarbone. Once it's in place, we can put the chemo in and take blood out without having to stick you in the arm every time."

I'm still pretty stressed, but here's an opening that I'm not about to miss.

"Well, hell, Thad. You're gonna install a bio-port. Why didn't you just come right out and say so?"

"A bio-port," he repeats, not comprehending.

"Thad, ever go to the movies?"

"With my kids sometimes."

"Ever see David Cronenberg's *eXistenZ?*"

"Can't say as I have." He seems mildly curious.

"Well, if you had, you would have learned about bio-ports. The film is about people who play computer games in virtual reality, and in order to enter this reality they have to be fitted with inserts at the base of their spines. Then they can get plugged in to the virtual scene of computer games directly. But the neato part is when a grease-smeared auto mechanic, played by Willem Dafoe, implants a bio-port in the main character with a huge pneumatic drill usually used to remove lug nuts from truck wheels."

Thad's looking a bit dreamy here, but he's neither interrupting nor walking out, so I just push ahead.

"Now once the bio-port's in place, people go on living normally until they want to play some virtual game. Then, just like you'll do with my catheter, they just plug in and turn on. So Thad, you gonna use a tire-drill on me or what?"

"I think I'll stick you with my needle."

He's still with me, but barely.

"Well, whatever works. Listen, I've got a great idea. Suppose I make you a video clip of that scene where the Dafoe character installs the bio-port. It is a little graphic, but it's also technology at work. What's important for you here is the rhetorical potential of this scene."

I pause here, waiting to see what he'll do.

"The rhetorical potential," he repeats blankly.

"Here's the deal. Take me for example. I'm absolutely terrified to have you, even on your very best day—and how would I even *know* if it's your very best day?—jam a needle with some goddamned piece of plastic hanging on it into my chest! What you need, what *I* need, is some reassurance that things could be a lot worse. You with me here?"

I'm not so sure he is, but press on anyway.

"And so, when you get your patient prepped for this catheter thing, you say, 'Now before I begin, I want to show you how we used to do this procedure.' Then just run the clip. Trust me on this one. After that clip, your patient will be so traumatized that you can bypass the anesthetic—you *do* use an anesthetic, don't you Thad? Just give 'em a swig of hooch, tell 'em to bite down hard on their belt, and jam away."

For what seems a long time, he never moves. Then he snaps out of it. He smiles at no one in particular, shifts on his stool and, without saying anything, begins to fill out the form for the catheter procedure.

Damn! I must have misread him. I could have sworn he was with me. Maybe this trickster strategy doesn't work with the heavy hitters in Cancerland. Maybe I'm a bit out of touch with Thad's reality. Clearly, it must not be fun to be an oncologist. For every time he gets to say "I can cure this," he's probably forced to say something far less encouraging. I wince at my own insensitivity. About all I can do is watch him fill out my form, and even that isn't easy because I'm seeing it upside down. He scribbles something in each blank. Where he must describe the procedure itself, he starts to write something, pauses, looks away, thinking, looks back, and then, as if he's made some private decision that puts him at peace with himself, completes the description. It takes me a second to unscramble what he's written. In the blank, the one where he's supposed to describe the procedure, it says "Install bio-port."

I did it! Kicking and screaming, perhaps, I induced Thaddeus out of his professional world and into some mega-bizarre movie context with a weirder-than-weird professor, and he actually played along, at least a little. It was a trickster moment I was not about to forget.

A week later Janice and I are in the office where Thad installs bio-ports. The office itself feels more like an executive suite than an installation center. It's open, bright, cheery, with only the dentist-type chair bolted in one corner suggesting the possibility of darker things. I'm already rehearsing our bio-port talk so I can build on it, but am too anxious to be very creative. Besides, Thad isn't even here yet. But his assistant is, and as she busies herself making things ready, she explains the procedure to me, presumably to put my mind at ease.

Or perhaps Thad has prepped her on what to say just to get even with me. As things unfold, I come to believe she's either been tipped off or she is just naturally sadistic.

"You'll be sitting right here, Dr. Frentz," she begins innocently enough. "We'll tilt the chair back so that your head is slightly lower than the rest of your body."

"And why would that be?"

"So the veins in your chest will protrude a bit and Dr. Carlson can more easily locate the one he's looking for."

" I knew I shouldn't have asked."

I have a bad feeling about this woman and it's beginning to show.

"Now, when Dr. Carlson is ready," she continues as if I weren't even there, "we'll give you a little local anesthetic that will feel like a tiny bee sting."

She delivers this last line as though she were talking to a two-year-old.

"Then Dr. Carlson will insert a needle into the large vein just beneath your collar bone," she drones, "run the catheter down the vein next to your heart and lung . . . "

"Stop right there. I think I'm gonna hurl."

No response, not even a trace of a smile. I think maybe I should barf just to catch her attention.

". . . fix a plastic vein opener onto the surface, sew a flange onto the skin with two tiny sutures to hold the vein opener in place," she concludes never missing a beat. "Then we . . ."

"Hold it! I'm think I'm gonna pass out."

". . . will x-ray your chest to see if everything's where it should be."

"And if it is?" I jump in quickly, relieved that the torture talk is over.

"And if it is," she repeats with just a touch of irritation, "we'll be through with you."

"Which means I can go home?" I ask, knowing better, but interested now in what she will say.

"Which *means*," there's that edge again, "that you can go down to the chemotherapy lab for your first treatment."

"Lucky me, eh?"

"Yes, actually, lucky you."

What a barrel of laughs Nurse Ratched is. A magician too, for in less than two minutes, she's transformed my feeling-slightly-anxious into a full-blown scared-to-death.

Just as I'm wondering how I might drool on her a little, Thad walks in.

He looks different, bright, refreshed, almost bouncy. Then I remember that he's had a week off. I watch him closely. His eyes are sharp, focused. He looks ready. That makes one of us.

"Strip to the waist, my good man," he says far too cavalierly for my present mood.

I do as I'm told and hop right into the wonderful tilting chair. It buzzes and tilts back, just like it's supposed to. I hear snapping as Thad pulls on rubber gloves. Then he's fussing with something, and I feel icy cold on my chest.

"Ow. What's that?"

"Iodine."

"You don't think I'm sterile?"

"You will be soon."

Not bad. He's still with me.

"So, Thad, see any movies while you were away?"

"Yep. Took my kids to *My Dog Skip.*"

"Yeah, I remember that one. That's where the rabid St. Bernard kills most of the people in a small town, right? Bet your kids just loved it."

"That would be *Cujo.*"

"Oh yeah, right. Catch *eXistenZ*?"

"Nope."

"Then how the hell are you gonna do this procedure?"

"Like Smith-Barney used to do investments. The old-fashioned way."

"Ouch. What are you doing now?"

"Shaving off some of your masculinity, so I can see what I'm doing."

"I like that. Seeing is good. New syringe, I hope?"

"Fairly new. All right. Now I need to tell you what could happen," and he begins reciting the medical profession's version of my Miranda rights.

"I could pop a lung, although I never have. Or I could put the catheter into an artery instead of a vein, in which case your blood would purify the chemo instead of the other way around. But that's never happened, either. Or I could . . . "

"Thad, you miserable dickwad! Don't you remember *anything* from medical school? Arteries are red, veins are blue—it's the oxygen–carbon dioxide interchange or something like that. You gotta keep this basic shit straight, man."

"You're right, of course. But there was just so much to remember. Arteries red, veins blue. Go for the blue. OK, I got it. Now, here comes the local."

"Local wha . . . Ouch! Feels like a goddamned bee sting."

"And the honey comes later."

"That would be a lame metaphorical reference to your poison, right?"

"That would be a lame metaphorical reference to your cure, right."

"Oh, right! Now, tell the truth. My cure is some thick sludge scooped out of a toxic waste dump with the larger impurities removed, right? And you're gonna put this stuff into my precious bodily fluids in hopes that it kills my cancer faster than it kills me. Is that about it?"

"That's about it."

Before I can follow this up, he backs away, snapping off the rubber gloves.

"You're through here. Let's get you off to x-ray and see if I've still got the touch."

Fast, and almost painless. Thad whipped through the entire procedure somewhere between a "bee sting" and an "x-ray." I'm pretty impressed. He tilts the chair back up.

"Oh, by the way, the real reason we tilt this chair back is to keep you from passing out." I don't think he's kidding. I glance down hesitantly at my chest. On the right side, just below my collarbone, is some tape and a small tube. I stand up cautiously, wondering if I might pass out. And then all hell breaks loose.

Just as I'm testing my sea legs, Thad jumps back, gets a manic look in his eyes, and says to Janice, with a dead-on Colin Clive accent: "There! I am Dr. Frankenstein and he is my monster. Away with him."

Poor Thad has no way of knowing how well I can play in Frankenstein's world. Janice and I had recently completed a book on the Frankenstein complex in films. I not only know the story very well but also have memorized large portions of the dialogue. And so, in my own very best Boris Karloff rasp, I give him the monster's retort, compliments of Mary Shelley:

> Remember that I am thy creature; I ought to be thy Adam, but
> am rather the fallen angel, whom thou drivest from joy for no
> misdeed. Everywhere I see bliss, from which I alone am irrevo-
> cably excluded. I was benevolent and good; misery made me a
> fiend. Make me happy, and I shall be virtuous. (84)

He shrinks back against the wall in mock horror.

"Out, fiend!" he cries. "You are not yet finished. You must return to my lab-*or*-a-tory for more work before virtue might again be a balm for your wretchedness."

No doubt convinced that she's in the presence of madness, Nurse Ratched obsessively stacks and restacks piles of little paper pill cups. To hell with her and all the Nurse Rat-Shits in the world, my wolf says. Let them bask humorlessly in a world of sheep constructed by medical shepherds. Thad and I have better places to go and more important things to do. We're living in film contexts this time, where I can ridicule Thad, he can make fun of me, all the while, back there on planet earth, he is doing what he needs to do. Savage the structure, save the face. Words to live by, I hope.

CHAPTER 10

Shepherd Tales

My chief concern is that our educational system does not focus on the inner lives of students or help them to acquire the self-understanding that is the basis for a satisfying life. Nor . . . does it provide the safe and nurturing environment that people need in order to grow.

Jane Tompkins
A Life in School: What the Teacher Learned

It's only fitting, I suppose, to have recovered my trickster within the Ass Festival. Historically, there really was such an event, a comic reversal of high church dogma in which the great unwashed and church officialdom often shared equally (Jung, *Four* 139–40). Without pressing the analogy too far, medical specialists are today's techno-gods, just as their clerical ancestors were once honored as emissaries of a more spiritual deity. So, when I invited my physicians and medical technicians to play with me in those liminal contexts, I was re-enacting an ancient ritual designed to keep a check on that annoying human tendency to make ourselves into gods. Players on the lower end of ass festivals employ humor, the central rhetorical strategy used by self-conscious tricksters, to break rules and disrupt order. Having just done that, I was feeling pretty puffed-up over my own rites of the rectum. But my pride was short-lived.

My first reality check came about when I read how some Marxist-oriented academicians mistrust the political consequences of "carnival," a more general name for structure-bending rites overseen by tricksters, because while comic ridicule may be cathartic for the disempowered, it rarely alters existing power structures. As Lewis Hyde puts it:

> Especially in highly ordered and hierarchical societies, carnival reinforces the status quo because . . . it provides the exceptions that prove the rules. We may laugh at men dressed as women, or greasy food eaten at the alter, but when the laugher ends, the normal patterns return all the more solidly. Carnival is, after all, officially sanctioned and clearly contained. The powers that be are in on the game; they give it space in the town square . . . and they control its timing. . . . Mocking but not changing the order of things, ritual dirt-work operates as a kind of safety value, allowing internal conflicts and nagging anomalies to be expressed without serious consequences. (187)

In one sense, the Marxists are right. I never did seriously disrupt the structure of the medical community. Doctors and technicians, from Heather to Thad, sanctioned and even played along with my transgressions, probably as a compassionate way to diffuse my anxieties. But, as far as I know, our comic interludes never changed the rigid hierarchy of the medical community in which I was immersed.

In another sense, these materialist critiques are wrong. Expecting carnival to destroy hierarchy altogether seems like a leftover Marxist ideal. For those who take the political potential of comic critique seriously, the rhetorical goal of such transgressions is *never* to obliterate structures, but only to reconfigure them into less rigid forms of social organization. Throughout the medical episodes, my own purpose was to create an imaginary setting with a new set of roles and rules in which I could preserve my humanity, all the while accepting the treatment offered by the medical specialists. In retrospect, I don't think those forms of carnival were merely cathartic acts. I believe that they functioned, at least to some degree, to humanize me in their eyes. If, through such humorous exchanges, the medical professionals came to see patients more as subjects and less as objects, then everybody won, even within the admittedly stratified confines of the medical community. That seems right. Perhaps I can allow a bit of coyote pride to seep back into my psyche. Marxists do not have the last word on trickster rites, after all.

But Janice may have. Feeling pretty cocky again, I run the argument by Janice.

"So, what do you think?" I ask, confidently.

"Well, it's a solid argument, but it's not going to get you out of the woods."

"What do you mean?"

"If I'm tracking you right here, you're moving towards an analogical argument that goes something like: 'What I did with those medical specialists is what I can now do with my academic colleagues.' Is that right?"

"Yeah, I guess that's where I'm heading. What's wrong with that?"

"Everything. There's just no connection between your doctors and your colleagues."

An absolute deal breaker.

"Huh?" I stall.

"Think about it," she instructs. "You respect your doctors because they have lots of technical know-how that you lack and need. But you *disrespect* most of your colleagues because you think, right or wrong, that you've forgotten more about the field of Communication than they'll ever know. Isn't that right?"

She knows it is.

"Moreover, your trickster is how you *begin* relationships. You've said earlier that when you get to know people, that voice almost always gives way to the sheep, if you like and respect people, or to the wolf, if you don't. You've been in this department now for—what?—over seventeen years. You still think playing the trickster is a viable option?"

"Probably not," I say dejectedly. I'm stuck now, with no place to go. Janice waits, allowing the despondency to sink in.

"Just because the analogy doesn't work," she continues hopefully, "doesn't mean something else won't."

"Right now I can't see what that might be."

She thinks a bit, and then adds, "Maybe it's time you stopped speaking like an animal."

"What?" I say, feeling attacked again.

"I didn't say that quite right. Up to here, your voices have all been identified with animals; coyote for your conscious trickster, wolf for the unconscious version, and sheep for your ultra-dependency. Isn't that right?"

"Sure, so what?"

"So it might be helpful to think back to times when you spoke and acted like a human; in Pirsig's terms, like a shepherd."

"Like a shepherd," I repeat dumbly.

"Sure. Remember what Art Bochner said to you once?"

"Art said lots of things to me."

"He said 'You still have the need to be funny.'"

"He did?"

"Don't stall. You know damned well he did."

"So, what's your point?"

"My point (and Art's point too) is that being funny, the staple of your trickster, keeps you in an adolescent, outsider role. As long as you limit yourself to those animals, even in fronting the coyote you undercut your own need for respect and influence, and then blame your colleagues for not respecting your latent genius. I *know* that as a professor you speak and act in other ways. My guess is that you're a pretty good shepherd, but you don't want to look at that because to do so would mean that you might have to grow up."

"Do I have to pay you for this?"

"As Ronald Reagan once said, 'There you go again,'" she counters. "Since you're not stuck bad enough to read anything that might help you right now, why don't you reflect on some shepherd acts where you liked what you did?"

"Do I have to?" I whine.

"Oh, hell no. Why don't you just blow me off and keep acting like a child?"

She's taking no prisoners today.

Much to my surprise, when I worked at it a little, some shepherd tales began to emerge. In 1995 I was president of our southern regional communication association. It was the highest position of authority I'd ever held. I loved it, and I think I was loved for it. Clearly, part of that affection came from my comedy routines. I was told that during my tenure I violated almost every rule of parliamentary procedure known to humankind. In part that was because I didn't know what most of the rules were, but in larger part it was because following the rules made those pompous official meetings feel like death marches. I was in trickster's heaven! I was also told that I'd crafted my transgressions with enough ingenuity and flair that even the most stalwart defenders of Roberts and his *Rules* were never seriously offended.

This presidency was more to me than just a public forum for coyote. Several years earlier, I was at a convention dinner with close friends when the presidency idea first came up.

"So, Frentz," one began, "I'm on the nominating committee for next year and we need someone to run for second vice-president. How about you?"

The entire table erupted in laughter. Apparently, my reputation had preceded me.

"How much will you pay me to run against whomever you really want to win?" I retorted.

"No, you'd win. Everybody in the region knows you. You have name recognition."

"Well, so would Jack Kevorkian," a supporter interjected.

"I don't think so," I began bailing, sensing a little too much seriousness.

"You'd get to give the speech," Janice tossed out not-so-innocently.

Hmmm. I *would* get to give the speech. The Presidential Address to the entire convention—to 300, maybe 400 people, all in one place, at the same time, all listening to me. That was mighty seductive to an old rhetor who had never had a public forum for his ideas.

"So," I asked in my best don't-give-a-shit manner, "what would I have to do?"

"Virtually nothing," snapped the nominating committee person, suddenly sensing victory where a moment ago there wasn't even a contest. "Just agree to run, write a three-paragraph vision statement for the monthly newsletter, and wait to be crowned."

Well, I thought, why not? What's the absolute worst thing that could happen? I'd get two votes, right? Janice's and mine. At least I *think* Janice would support me. At least I'd have a life-long arsenal of quips to use at future conferences. That wouldn't be such a bad trade-off.

"Oh hell, why not?" I blurted.

So I ran and won. Most important, I got to deliver the Presidential Address.

When I reread that speech, I'm surprised at how much I still like it. I'm even more surprised at how shepherd-like it is. It's entitled, "The Unbearable Darkness of Seeing," a fairly transparent spin off of Milan Kundera's novel, *The Unbearable Lightness of Being*. In it I speak openly about our deepest wounds as an academic field, about our discipline's shadow—that we have no unified subject matter, no indigenous methods of inquiry, no acclaimed theories or theorists, and no credibility among cognate disciplines or university administrators. Is it any wonder that we have such a massive inferiority complex? Then, guided by Ursula Le Guin's *A Wizard of Earthsea* (Le Guin), I wonder whether our most profound weaknesses could turn into our most enduring strengths. In her tale, Ged, a gifted young wizard-in-training, impulsively releases his own shadow, which proceeds to hunt and haunt him throughout his life. I show how Communication, like Ged, has been diminished and persecuted throughout history by its own demons, first by the philosophers and later by minions of the social sciences.

The key move, for Communication, as for Ged, then, is to stop running, turn around, and face and embrace the shadow as much devalued parts of ourselves. If we could ever be comfortable as an interdisciplinary field of study, we would be uniquely positioned to reconnect other fragmented and estranged academic units into a more unified and politically potent university community. If we could ever come to terms with being made up of fragments of knowledge originating in other scholarly disciplines, we might generate theoretical insights by metaphorically fusing these seemingly dissimilar fragments into common points of view. I concluded with:

> It is time, I believe—long past time—for us to follow Ged's example. Let us speak our shadow's name. Let us reach out for its dark self. Let us hold it close to our heart. Let us, in other words, endure the unbearable darkness of seeing as a prelude to the unbearable lightness of being. (19)

I received a standing ovation. One of the grand women of Performance Studies made her way through the well-wishers and said, with tears in her eyes, "You, sir, are a poet." It was my finest public moment, and it wasn't funny at all.

I keep cycling back to this account of my speech and I'm not sure why. I know part of it is that I'm not completely happy with the way it sounds. I'm afraid that in order to get the ideas across I've slipped back into sheep speak. I've been tweaking it endlessly, trying to exorcise that sound and preserve the more accessible prose that better reflects how I want to be heard. But there's more going on than just the sound of my voice. I'm struggling with this speech because, in many ways, it is a bona fide shepherd statement. Throughout the whole address, I'm pushing—pushing really hard—for accepting fragmentation as a prelude to some greater form of wholeness. The value of interconnectedness is literally stitched into every phrase, every argument, every citation, every figure. This speech was, I now think, my attempt to share my vision of the field as a *person*, not through one of my animal voices.

I finally stopped tinkering with that irksome paragraph and asked Janice to read it. I thought it was good, and wanted some spousal praise and celebration for my efforts.

"How's that?" I ask, with a bit too much self-satisfaction.

"It's wonderful," she affirms. "It really is. Brings back all of the emotional intensity of that moment. You've really caught the mood well. I really like all that, but . . ." she hesitates.

"But what?"

"Well, I hate to be picky, but you know what really jumps out at me?"

"No, but you're gonna tell me, right?"

"What jumps out at me is that you're still performing, still the center of attention."

"Well Jesus, Janice! It's a goddamned presidential address! Of *course* I was performing. What did you expect me to do, email everybody?"

"Now don't go cranky on me. All I'm saying is that this particular moment, while clearly not based on your trickster, sheep, or wolf, is one in which you were *the* central authority figure. As I need not remind you, times when you have been that empowered are pretty few and far between. So while that speech was clearly a shepherd tale, I'm wondering if it was, as you used to say, 'a statistical rare event'?"

She sees that I'm ripe for another gentle push.

"What we need," she continues, and I greatly appreciate the third-person plural pronoun here, "are some times when you spoke like a shepherd but when you were not in the public eye. And when, also, you liked who you were. Can you think of some times like that?"

"Sure, when I'm asleep. But it's pretty hard to build off that," I grumble, not giving up without a few well-chosen sulks.

"I was thinking more of how you work with students you like," she says ignoring me.

"Oh that sounds exciting," I sulk. "Maybe I could run through a few degree checks, explain my reasoning on a few exam questions, design a hypothetical schedule of classes for a Communication major. That ought to turn readers on."

"It sounds like you're still all hung up on shepherds having to be the center of attention. Give this a try. I'll bet there have been some moments with particular students in which you liked who you were *because* you helped them blossom on their own. I can think of lots of examples right off the bat, but *you've* got to think of them because they become important only if you like who you were in them."

"This isn't going to be easy."

"Hard things never are," she says. "Why don't you start with Fred Williams? After all, he was the surrogate father who shepherded you into the academic fold. Maybe you learned a few shepherd tricks from him."

Janice was right. Once I thought of Fred, I was on my way again.

It's 1969 and I'm about to receive the "Fred Williams Lecture." I'm working very hard on my dissertation. Fred sees that everybody works very hard on their dissertation. A few make it, a few more don't. I'm going to be one who does. I really push, but I slip-slide a bit too. I nearly kill myself Mondays through Fridays, but then on Saturdays and Sundays, when Fred thinks I should get the most done because I don't have to teach, I sneak out of Madison, drive eighty-five miles back to Oshkosh, shoot ducks, and spend romantic interludes with my high school sweetheart. My not-so-secret ambition is to get a job at the University of Wisconsin, Oshkosh, marry Ms. Sweetheart, and hunt forever. Fred knows this and it eats at him (I almost wrote "at his soul," but I don't want to make any rash assumptions here). But he also knows how much I respect his support and trust. So late one night, after he's sure I'm worn down from dissertating, he decides to change my life.

"So, Brain Damage. What are you up to after you get this thing done?"

Caught completely unawares, I make the same mistake I'll make with Janice many years later. I tell the truth.

"You know me, Cap. I'll probably just head back home, try to catch on at the local college, hunt, and hang out."

He stiffens, leans forward, gives me a look that would freeze lava, and starts his (in)famous speech: "Like hell you will! Now, you listen to me. I don't waste my time with minor-league ballplayers. Never have. Academic life's too short and brutal to waste time on those who'd rather waste time themselves. I tease you with all that 'Brain Damage' talk, but hear me clearly: I wouldn't be messing with you if I didn't believe that you could play in the major leagues. You are going to be a first-rate scholar. You got that? *You can play in the majors!*"

I got it. For the first time, I even began to believe that I might have what it takes to be an academic. Fred, however, was not finished.

"I'll be goddamned if I'm going to let you piss your life away hunting ducks, having kids, and kissing your old man's ass. Communication has nurtured you from a snotty-nosed ex-soldier into a first-rate scholar. It's time for you to give something back to Communication. You got that, BD?"

I'm stunned, not sure whether to feel elated or deflated.

"So, what do you think I should do?" I ask, a bit dependently.

"Go to California. Get as far away from here as you can. My old PhD advisor works at a pretty good university out there. I could probably get you in. Want me to try?"

"Any ducks in California?"

"None that you can hunt. You'll be too busy writing and making a name for yourself."

That was it, the Fred Williams' Lecture. He had me, but I had something too—his unabashed commitment to me as an academician.

I never forgot that lecture. It was my first lesson in how to be a good shepherd. I also never forgot that I was not Fred Williams. Whereas I gave his late-night litany to a select few over the years (with mixed results, I might add), my version of his lecture was another performance ritual. What wasn't performance, what Fred really gave me beneath his own bravado, and what I've tried to give back to promising students, was his unswerving trust and belief in me as a teacher and scholar. I think Janice wants me to go to where my own involvement with students comes more from listening to what *they* want to do than from my telling them what *I* want them to do. I guess it's still fashionable these days for high profilers to turn graduate students into clones and acolytes. But that's never been a big deal with me, even as a medium profiler, because I've always found the impulse behind such practices to be driven more by self-promotion than by concern for students' well-being. I'm sure my history figures in here, because I've spent a goodly part of my own career trying to wean myself from theories, methods, and ideas that were more valued by others than they ever were by me.

Alyssa, who's clearly not your ordinary student, drifts into my office one day in the fall of 1997, sitting down with a bit too much self-assured casualness.

"Hi, I'm Alyssa. You're my graduate advisor. You ever go to science fiction conventions?"

I glance up to see a young woman with bright blue eyes, flaming red hair, a nice batch of freckles, and wearing early grunge. No face metal or tattoos that I can see.

"No, Alyssa, I don't go to science fiction conventions, but I do sometimes write about science fiction films. Does that count?"

I'm opting for a quick dose of professorial condescension designed to put her in her place. I am not, after all, totally immune to hierarchy. But it never even registers.

"I guess. At least you know the genre. But the real rush is to go as a series character—you know, like Darth Vader—and to show up in costume. William and I often make our own . . ."

"William?" I interrupt, hoping that she'll come up for air.

"My hub-bud. I often make costumes for us. We stay in character the entire time. Just hang out, dress like the characters, talk like the characters, and even improvise as a situation might demand. That way we get some neat autographs, meet some important people connected to the series, and do some serious networking that might someday land us a part-time job on a series set. That would be just *tres* cool. William's a great scriptwriter. He did some minor revision work for a couple of *Babylon 5* episodes. To defer the cost of attending these things—some years we go to fifteen or twenty conventions—Russell and I collect and sell rare one-of-a-kind sci-fi memorabilia. Say, would you be at all interested in the original light saber that Mark Hamill used in *Star Wars*?"

All of this pours out in what Tom Farrell once called the "oh yeah, and another thing" pattern of organization.

"Ummm . . . not today," I jump in. "But back in the here and now, how might I help you with your degree program?"

I up my drudge factor, trying hard to find a subject we can share.

"Oh that. Yeah . . . well—as I guess you can tell already—I'm just too weird to be anything other than an academic."

"Gosh, I wouldn't have guessed that at all."

"I already know all of your graduate requirements. I have a photographic memory. It comes in handy sometimes. I blew the bloomers off the GREs last summer—scored, I forget, 1480 or something. Never studied at all, just walked in, sat down, and swallowed 'em whole. The questions are so goddamned predictable. So, anyway, I want to do the thesis option, and I was thinking . . ."

". . . that maybe you should take a few classes first?" I am hoping that a little spontaneous cloze procedure might help keep us on track here.

"Sure, that too, but I was thinking about the thesis option and . . ."

". . . and you already have an idea or two, am I right here?"

"Yeah actually, you are. See I'm an ecofeminist, and a member of the local Wicca chapter, and I might want to . . ."

"The local 'whacca' chapter?"

"Wicca—you know, witches—women who worship goddesses more than gods. Definitely *not* witches in the male-defined Hollywood sense of wart-covered, perverted, blood-sucking, child-molesting old crones that need a good burning every now and then. I might want to do a thesis about witches."

From "Hi, I'm Alyssa" to a "thesis about witches" in five free-floating moves. I'm in way over my head here, I'm thinking. Just stay calm. She will, in all likelihood, levitate out of your office any second now. But she doesn't and, as we pause for a moment and just look at each other, I'm beginning to wonder how—or even if—I can ever really contact planet Alyssa.

I do eventually make contact with Ms. Alyssa, here and there, in fits and starts, over that extended and very strange period of time known as her degree program. Once we tacitly agree that one of us is most likely an extant species, we stumble our way into a relationship of mutual care and fragile trust, affirmed only sporadically by a quirky set of conversational non sequiturs. As she once did the GREs, Alyssa swallows our entire graduate program whole. In the process, she introduces me, mostly against my better judgment, to the bizarre world that she and William inhabit. It's a liminal realm suspended precariously between neurosis and madness. I get to see Alyssa in her Princess Leia outfit from *Return of the Jedi*, and I'm forced to see William as the head-in-a-jar from *Dune*.

As her thesis deadline looms, Alyssa and I struggle with her prospectus. She writes like she thinks, and she thinks like she talks, and she talks in fragments about fragments of everything, all at once. Her one area of academic consistency, the one she never strays too far from, is women's issues. Granted, her take on these issues places her (how would I say it in science speak?) more than two standard deviations from any mean, but they are women's issues nonetheless. By happy coincidence, at that time I too am involved in feminist theories—mostly French, primarily radical—and, given Alyssa's penchant for the stranger than strange, I figure this is a match that might work. If I can only get her to use some aspect of feminist theory to say something novel and intelligible about women, perhaps a thesis may yet be forthcoming. But I can't get her to go there, no matter how hard I try. So I call her in and cut right to the chase.

"So, Wicca Mistress of Darkness, how's the thesis stand?"

"On its ass."

"Know why?"

"Nope. Thought you might. You're the big Kahuna on these things."

"I've no clue," and this time I'm not lying.

She's silent, a very bad sign because Alyssa is never silent. I don't know what to say either, so we both just sit there stewing. Then, seemingly out of nowhere, I have an idea, a good-shepherd moment.

"All right—quick, without thinking—what do you hate most about your general thesis area?"

"Those fucking French feminists you made me read." This as if I've just jabbed her with a cattle prod.

"Again quick, without thinking, why?"

"Because their power as women is based on their writing like men. If you 'theorize' women, you're doing to women exactly what men have always done to women—and anything else they wanted to colonize and control—putting them in nice little categories arranged in nice little hierarchies. All those radical French bitches in smelly jockstraps."

Now we're cooking and my lines are coming easier.

"All right, once more now—still, quick, without thinking—what do you want to write about?"

"Starhawk."

"An Indian or a bird?"

"Neither, racist pig! She's an ecofeminist who just ass-slaps all those father-obsessed French floozies."

"And how does she do that?"

"By historicizing women through feminine spiritualities. She recovers what most people never see, namely, how women can find themselves through repressed remnants of Goddess religions, rather than sitting around passively while the patriarchy builds them in its own image."

"So one more time, without thinking, how would you go about studying this Starhawk person?"

"Not the way you'd want me to. Look, like it or not, you're still all hung up on 'method'—most guys are. But a 'method' is a male-generated distancing device that takes me out of what I need to get into. So if I use some formal 'method' in the standard academic sense, I'm undercutting what I want to do even as I do it. I'd like to just immerse myself, as a woman, in Starhawk's texts and see what I might find about being a woman. Can I do that?" she asks hopefully.

"Absolutely."

"All right!" she makes me high-five her. "I'll have chapter 1 in ten days."

She does, too, followed quickly by all the rest. It's a wonderful piece of work, radical, innovative, rigorous, and written with just the right blend of spiritual wisdom and political outrage. I've come to appreciate my place in Alyssa's world. I think I let her become more fully herself by listening, empathizing, coaxing, being those things my mother once taught me how to do, but now doing them without compromising myself in the process. As Fred Williams once did for me, I now do for Alyssa. That feels like progress.

I know now that I have spoken as a shepherd, and that I like the sound of that voice more than I thought I would. I know too that I spoke mostly as a temporary dignitary or as a mentor to students. The real conundrum here involves my professional colleagues, the alpha-shepherds in any department and in my field. After more than thirty years of nonproductive relationships with most of them, is it even realistic to consider changing practices that seem to be set in stone? I don't feel at all confident about this, but it's time to crawl back into the trenches and see what's going on.

CHAPTER 11

Trials in the Trenches

Morons. I've got morons on my team.

Percy Garris

Butch Cassidy and the Sundance Kid

Obsessing about how—or even whether—to include this chapter pushed me up against what Pirsig's Phaedrus confronted in *Zen*, namely, the horns of a dilemma. If I remain silent, I'm impaled on the horn that tacitly reaffirms the very structures I think need changing, while, if I speak, I'm run through on the other horn that labels me a trouble maker. In the novel, Phaedrus attacked his dilemma straight on and went mad. Being crazy enough already, I'm opting for one of the rhetorical moves Phaedrus considered but didn't pursue, namely, the "between the horns" strategy that says, in effect, the dilemma will disappear if I enlarge the context in which it appears (207). Thus, in what follows, I craft a narrative by stitching together three episodes drawn from departments in three different universities. My intention is to focus attention on the disfunctionality of certain structural rules and not on the particular personalities of those who generate and protect them.

After more than thirty years in the profession, I've learned a few things about departmental structures. For the most part, they are constructed, not by the written pronouncements found in academic officialdom, but by less formal, unwritten rules that evolve over time, rigidify with practice, eventually come to be seen as "natural," and are usually referenced obliquely by expressions like, "This is how we do things around here." Like all rules, these are a mixed bag. On the up side, they specify codes of academic civility and guide departmental activities toward collective ends. On the down side, those who benefit most from these rules are the authority figures who make them up; if those in power do their jobs right, the rules both legitimize and reproduce their power structures. Because those who benefit most from the rules are seldom motivated to change them, that thankless task inevitably falls to someone else. Theoretically, rule changing is the centerpiece of a trickster's job description. But departments, I've also learned, don't work theoretically, and authority figures are not particularly fond of tricksters. And vice versa.

I have been coordinator of the basic course in Communication for several departments. This is the story of one of them. Coordinating the basic course is a big job, involving selecting a textbook, developing an overall course syllabus, working out daily lesson plans, coordinating media for multiple classrooms, and supervising anywhere from ten to twenty-five graduate teaching assistants who vary significantly in motivation, experience, and teaching ability. I was savvy enough to know that, as coordinator, I could perform some of these tasks independently but had to clear others with the powers-that-be. The trick was knowing which were which. I scheduled a meeting with my chair.

"So, chief," I begin, "what can I do and what can't I do as honcho of this class?"

"You can do just about anything you want," he says, unhelpfully.

"Can you clarify 'just about'?" I push, trying to get an explicit interpretation of the operable rules governing my position.

"Sure. If you want to change the text or the basic philosophy of the course, you'll need to run that by the undergraduate committee. That's because this class is not only our major cash cow but it also functions as a college-wide service course in which other units have a vested interest."

"That makes sense. But what about supervising TAs, modifying lessons plans, stuff like that?" I ask.

"You can change any of that, as you like. If you had to consult me or the undergraduate committee on everything, the coordinator position would be a redundancy, wouldn't it?"

"It would," I agree. "Thanks." That wasn't so hard, I think. All I had to do was ask. But, as I was soon to discover, it *was* hard, and having asked didn't help at all. I didn't change anything at first; I just hung out, kept my eyes and ears peeled, and took some notes. What I discovered was that some things worked and others didn't. As coordinator, I locked in on what didn't. For one thing, the TAs seemed paralyzed by endless ticky-tacky rules that specified everything from classroom attire to teaching postures. For another, every class period was micromanaged, right down to the exact wording of specific examples. For a third, there was no mechanism for helping TAs handle all of those relational issues that arise in classrooms when instructors are only slightly older and more experienced than their students. In these straightjackets, TAs became objects that moved, not subjects who acted (Burke, "Dramatism" 445–52). These strictures seemed well within the purview of things my chair said I could change, so I changed them.

I tossed out the dress code, saying only that everyone had to wear underwear (Vivian Polk notwithstanding), and that no one could teach standing on his or her head. Good trickster talk. Next, I softened all those rigid lesson plans by creating general outlines for each class but encouraging TAs to develop their own examples, digress if and when they felt it necessary, and be concerned only to cover the main points on the day they were assigned. We spent wonderful hours brainstorming ideas and examples for the new TAs—who were struggling, as all new TAs do, to stay one chapter and one period ahead of their students. Then, like a good shepherd, I added some structure. I scheduled weekly meetings to hear and, wherever possible, diffuse relational problems in the classroom. "For the first time, I feel heard and understood," one TA told me shortly after I instigated these changes.

The TAs and I quickly bonded into a close-knit group. This was not communitas, in Victor Turner's sense; it was still a structure, but it was much looser than the one I inherited. I started to write that I was the good shepherd and they were my willing, and very appreciative, sheep, but that metaphor would have been one-sided. For the department power brokers, an entirely different metaphor was emerging, one that cast me as the alpha wolf teaching my pups to snarl and nip at the heels of the shepherds. Both metaphors were probably correct, but I wonder if I was even aware of this other view. I probably was, but, being caught up in the adoration of the TAs, I didn't care that much. Tricksters need love too! I see now how my bonding with the TAs established a dynamic that I still play out to this day. I become much more open, vulnerable, and accessible to select students than to most faculty, because (usually feeling power-down and somewhat isolated from my colleagues) I identify much more closely with students than I do with faculty. It's a problem. I remember once, when attending a wedding reception for a graduate student, Janice and I automatically sat with the students. One glanced mischievously over his shoulder at the faculty table and asked, "Are you two going to sit with us or with the grown-ups over there?"

Over time, a rift developed between me and the TAs, on the one hand, and the faculty on the other. I had felt empowered as coordinator of this course; I'm pretty sure the TAs felt empowered too. But some of the faculty probably didn't, because underlings were now calling into question many of their long-standing policies. If you want to reduce a person's or an institution's power over you, reduce your own dependency upon that person or that institution for things you value and need (Emerson). If the TAs could get more of what they valued and needed from me and had to depend less on other faculty for those things, then the faculty's power over them was diminished (but mine was increased). If the faculty could not justify the procedures for controlling the TAs, then those procedures should be changed (and I was around to help with that). At the time, it all seemed simple and straightforward to me. Take a rigid, oppressive structure, loosen and reconfigure it, and you get a better structure. Having asked my chair about these very issues, I felt legitimated to make the changes I made. I remembered Richard Emerson, but I should have remembered what Jock Ewing said to his son Bobby on the defunct television series *Dallas*: "Nobody *gives* you power, Bobby. Power is something you *take*."

In less than a year, my chair takes back what he had given.

"I'm hearing some pretty negative things about how you're running the basic course," he begins, after calling me in for "a chat."

"Oh? What seems to be the problem?" I ask innocently.

"*Problems*, in the plural. I hear you've not only changed the entire class but you're also blaming the rest of the faculty for everything the TAs don't like," he says with an accusatory edge.

"That's simply not true," I say calmly. "I've only changed what wasn't working, and only those things that I cleared with you a year ago."

"Well, you apparently misunderstood what I cleared for you to change."

Here's that damned discretionary thing thrown up in my face. In a context like this, when a chair tells a faculty member that he or she "misunderstood me," that generally means something like, "I'm changing the rules to get things back to the way they were and put you back in your place."

"I'm spending far too much of my time fielding your colleague's complaints about how you're running things," he continues. "I don't have time for that, so I'm going to replace you as basic course coordinator. Actually, it may be a blessing in disguise because you should have more time to do your research." This last bon bon comes coated with icy condescension.

Why were my chair and, by extension, select colleagues, so threatened by what I had done? In structural terms, I didn't see—or preferred not to see—that to reinterpret *any* rules that would realign the power dynamics in an academic unit was a no-no, particularly with those who felt the changes usurped their authority. For me, of course, those old power alignments had caused the problems in the first place. To ignore them would be to affirm them, and tricksters don't operate that way. Were there other, more "rhetorically sensitive" ways to go about these changes? Of course. Was I aware of any of them at the time? Of course not.

By the time I assumed this position as director of graduate studies, I'd already learned one valuable lesson in departmental survival: Consider how *what you do* affects others, rather than how *what others say you can do* might affect them. With that aphorism in mind, I hunkered down and reviewed the policies, written and tacit, about the way directors of graduate studies were to conduct their business. Clearly, one priority was to rank graduate students who applied for financial support as teaching assistants, and then pass my rankings along to the graduate committee for final approval. The criteria used in the ranking were crucial, so I studied them carefully. On the surface, they seemed clear, fair, and unremarkable: undergraduate grade point average (GPA); several letters of recommendation from the faculty; and a "goals statement," intended, I presumed, to show how well applicants could write.

Looking a bit more closely, I noticed that GPAs were taken at face value. It didn't seem to matter whether a student carried a demanding undergraduate load or a more leisurely one; a 3.85 GPA was always ranked higher than a 3.18 GPA. This made sense numerically, but I'd been around long enough to know that some students discover how to finesse the difficult courses to pad their GPAs. On a hunch, I reviewed the undergraduate transcripts of our current TAs, and I found that in many cases their undergraduate course work did not appear terribly demanding. This suggested to me that "raw" GPAs might not be a valid indicator of who should and should not receiving TA funding.

I also discovered that more than 95 percent of the current TAs had been in-state Communication majors. At first I figured that, since I wasn't working at an Ivy League school, most of our TA applicants *would* be in-state majors, but when I reviewed the applicants for the past five years that was not the case. We had numerous international student applicants, many with sterling credentials, who didn't make the cut. Some excellent out-of-state applicants were given little consideration. A few in-state applicants who did not major in Communication, but whose credentials far surpassed those of our best current TAs, fell by the wayside too.

I didn't like the looks of this. Why would these students, most with credentials superior to those of our current TA population, be passed over? As soon as I asked the question, the troubling answer was evident: because they lacked the "regional cultural background" thought necessary to relate well to the majority of our undergraduates. If that were true, these criteria created an insular, cultural homogeneity by ensuring that our TAs and their students shared the same cozy little worldview. I came to see that those seemingly innocent, straightforward criteria for selecting TAs were, in fact, a presumably unconscious means of denying cultural diversity. As a trickster, I had a bit of trouble with that.

So I made a few changes. I contacted the international students with the strongest credentials and began helping them navigate "the rhetoric of no" so often practiced in international student offices. Then I used some of my contacts to induce highly qualified undergraduates from around the country to pursue an MA in our department. My strategy went something like this: "If you send us some of your better undergraduates, we'll give them a first-rate MA and then send them back to you for their doctoral work." In a few cases, this actually worked. Finally, I massaged the GPAs, using 75 percent of grades from the general college requirements, and 25 percent from advanced Communication classes. Naturally, the rankings I submitted to the graduate committee using my "altered" criteria differed from those using the more traditional standards. Not too surprisingly, the graduate committee tossed my rankings aside, re-ranked the applicants using the old criteria, and never looked back. I had not, apparently, acted in accordance with "how things are done around here."

Having learned one hard lesson about departmental process, I was not about to blow off the powers-that-be again. This time, I drafted a formal proposal and submitted it to the graduate committee. I argued that we should require all TA applicants to take the Graduate Record Exam (GREs), and that these scores could be used as a crosscheck against GPAs in one of three ways. First, if a student combined high GREs with a high GPA, we could be confident of funding a superior student. Second, if a student had high GREs, but a low GPA, we may well be looking at an underachiever. As such, we would know in advance there was some risk in committing funding. Finally (and this was, of course, my not-so-hidden agenda), if a student had low GREs, but a high GPA, we might be dealing with an overachiever, or, in some cases, with an average student who had learned the art of taking undemanding undergraduate classes. Knowing these possibilities, we could act accordingly. The graduate committee was less than thrilled with my proposal.

Not long after that, my chair called me in.

"Tom, I'm getting some flak from the graduate committee on your ranking of TA applicants."

"Well, I have modified the criteria to give us a more diverse TA population," I admit.

"Diversity isn't the only thing we're after in our TA population."

"I know that, but if everything else is equal, isn't diversity important?"

"Of course it is, but the graduate committee tells me that everything else is not equal."

"Like what?" I ask, figuring I know what's coming.

"Like being able to relate to our undergraduate students. Over the years, we've found that our best TAs, those who are rated most highly by their students, are those who are well trained in the communication skills of our discipline. That's one reason why we tend to prefer our own undergraduate majors for our TAs."

There it is, I think. A slick little segue where "communication skills" stands for cultural homogeneity.

"But how do we assess the so-called communication skills of TA applicants?" I ask, already knowing his answer.

"We rely primarily on what our faculty says about them in their letters of recommendation," he affirms. "After all, our faculty knows our majors better than anyone, having taught them the very skills they will need in the classroom."

"But doesn't that give an unfair advantage to students who know our faculty? What about diversity of knowledge, superior abilities in related disciplines, cross-cultural and racial experiences?" I ask.

"I'm not saying those things aren't important," he says flatly, in a tone that suggests he's tired of sparring now, "but we've had pretty good luck doing it this way for quite some time," he says. "You ever hear the expression, 'If it ain't broke, don't fix it'?"

"I have," I say, "but I think some things *are* broke. I think too many applicants from other states, other countries, other races, and with other majors are not being given a fair shot at these assistantships. If you look at our current pool of TAs, they all look alike, dress alike, think alike, and act alike. Hell, they look like a herd of Stepford students," I add, with way too much wolf fang now showing.

He's quiet for a moment, and then come the words I've heard before.

"I guess we're pretty far apart on this TA thing. While I'm certainly sympathetic to your views, they simply do not reflect my own or those of the graduate committee. Given that, it might be better if somebody else were to coordinate our graduate program, somebody who's more in sync with departmental procedures."

There it is again. That insidious "This is how we do things around here" offered to cover up the real agenda, "Rules that sustain a given power structure will not be changed." For the second time, I'm forced to step down just after I've stepped up. I can't seem to speak with a voice that effectively changes structures I believe to be oppressive. Sheep speak gets me ignored, trickster talk gets me isolated, and wolf howls get me tossed off the mountain. If academia is the Church of Reason, I keep thinking, why do some people seem so goddamned unreasonable? Or *are* they? Am I the one who keeps pushing the envelope of reason beyond its academic limits? Thinking back on this episode, I see now (as I didn't then) how I backed my chair, and, by extension, the graduate committee, into a corner with my "I'm right and you're wrong" dichotomy, thereby creating their "dig-in-the-heels" defensiveness. Instead of breaking down oppositions, as I promised to do in the first chapter, I was creating them, and everybody was losing.

With these anxieties front and center, I'm more than ready for another breakfast table chat with Janice.

"I'm stuck now."

"I know," Janice says softly.

"How do you know?"

"Because you act stuck."

"What should I do?"

"You know what you should do."

"Write more?"

"Don't get cute. You know what you should do."

"Stop writing, right?"

"Stop writing, right."

"Then what?"

She doesn't respond to this right off, but sits back and looks out the window. After what feels like an hour, she turns to me and says carefully, "I think you need to stay in your stuckness for awhile. I know it's not pleasant being there, it never is, but if you leave too soon, you'll do nothing more than get caught up again in the same problem that put you there in the first place."

While I'm letting that sink in, she seems to drift off again, but I know better. Then she adds this: "It might be helpful to read—perhaps even write—about two things. Start by re-reading your own academic God figure, Pirsig, on the value of stuckness. Then try one of my God figures by reading Jung on 'the transcendent function,' his way to get unstuck. Then just loaf for a day, a week, maybe longer, and just give your unconscious time and space to play around with those two sets of meanings. I'll bet that in time you'll dream yourself up something important."

She knows that Pirsig will hook me in, and that, once hooked, I'll move on to Jung. She's also dead sure that only my unconscious can unravel this dilemma. I'm not really dead sure about anything right now, so I go back to Bob.

The section in question starts off simply enough: "Stuckness. That's what I want to talk about today" (272). Pirsig sets up a hypothetical case of mechanical stuckness, where a screw holding the side plate of a motorcycle engine in place breaks off inside the housing. But because this book works on multiple levels simultaneously, that's not the only form of stuckness Pirsig has in mind. He's also speaking about a relational stuckness between him and his son in the narrative, and an even deeper relational schism between him and his alter ego, Phaedrus, in his psyche. He could have been speaking of my department and me.

> This is the zero moment of consciousness. Stuck. No answer. Honked. Kaput. It's a miserable experience emotionally. You're losing time. You're incompetent. You don't know what you're doing. You should be ashamed of yourself. You should take the machine to a *real* mechanic who knows how to figure these things out. (273)

He goes on to exhaust the rational solutions for extracting the screw. Each failed attempt recycles him back into stuckness. Then this non-Western insight:

> Stuckness shouldn't be avoided. It's the psychic predecessor of all real understanding. An egoless acceptance of stuckness is a

key to understanding all Quality, in mechanical work, as in other endeavors. It's the understanding of Quality as revealed by stuckness which so often makes self-taught mechanics so superior to institute-trained men who have learned how to handle everything except a new situation. (279)

So I decide to take Pirsig's advice to heart and just sit tight. Well, I did read a little Jung while I was sitting.

Like Pirsig, Jung says that when our consciousness gets all stopped up and can't move forward, the best thing to do, perhaps the only thing to do, is nothing, just stay with the feelings and wait for a compensatory insight from the unconscious to break into awareness and change everything. He calls this breaking into awareness process "the transcendent function" (*The Portable Jung* 273–300). As I get it, this transcendent function works in the psyche much like a paradigm shift works in science. In science, a new paradigm doesn't so much negate what we thought we knew within the old paradigm as much as it re-contextualizes the knowledge in ways that radically alter what we thought it meant. Similarly, in the transcendent function, when unconscious meanings break into consciousness, our sphere of awareness changes so that the old meanings are understood in a new way. But neither new paradigms in science nor new frames of consciousness can be willed into existence, because willing itself occurs within the limited world views being transcended. So I just stayed stuck and waited for my unconscious to do what it's there to do, open up new ways of understanding.

As stucknesses go, this one hadn't been too terrible. It was bad sometimes, otherwise it wouldn't be stuckness, but for the most part I'd been doing the equivalent of going fishing. I slept late, jotted down my dreams whenever I remembered them, fertilized my roses, did odd jobs around the house, and, when the spirit moved me, edited the earlier parts of this story.

The next day, I went to see Larry Crandall, my doctor and long-time friend. I had been having some discomfort under my arm, and since lymph nodes are under there, and since I had an all-too-recent history of cancer in my lymph system, I didn't want to delay checking this out. I knew it would be a stressful visit, not only because of my escalating fears but also because I didn't have an appointment and, as a walk-in, I'd probably be left in Larry's waiting room interminably. On my way out the door, literally without looking or thinking, I grabbed a book. Only when I was sitting in the waiting room did I see that it was Arthur Frank's *At the Will of the Body*.

Leave it to me to take a cancer book to cheer me up while waiting to find out whether I still had cancer! I'd already read Frank's book several times, and had already cited it several times to help me through my cancer treatment. And so, somewhat bored, I just stood the book on end and let it fall open. It opened to a chapter entitled "The Struggle Is Not a Fight." I began to read. As if for the first time, I finally understood the distinction Frank was trying to make. He spoke about how he and his wife Cathie talked about cancer as a struggle, as living life during a war time, but never of cancer as the enemy:

> We never thought of "the cancer" as a thing to be fought. That would have personified it. . . . Cancer is not some entity separate from yourself. . . . The tumors may have been a painful part of me, they may have threatened my life, but they were still me. They were part of a body that would not function much longer unless it changed, but that body was still who I was. I could never split my body into two warring camps: the bad guy tumors opposed to the naturally healthy me. There was only one me, one body, tumors and all. Accepting that I was still one body brought me a great sense of relief. (84)

This time I got it. Just as Frank came to see that health and illness were not opposing forces at war but alternating states of his body, I came to see that my various academic personae were not warring complexes but alternating states of my psyche. In that waiting room, I began to let go of some of those oppositional ways of thinking and acting that had held me in thrall for far too long. It sounds pretty heady and abstract when I say it like this, but later the same day it would crystallize in, of all things, a feline form.

My arm was fine, no cancer recurrence. I was celebrating that evening, sitting on our front porch sipping a glass of white Zinfandel, waiting for Janice and watching our cat Mollie. She was focusing intently on a nice, plump, blue-tailed skink, her protein of choice in the summer, and paying me absolutely no mind. All of a sudden she stopped, almost in mid-stalk, spun on her haunches and looked directly into my eyes. Cat lovers will instantly understand this as a soul connection. I knew in an instant, although I didn't yet "know" in a way I could talk about, that something very important had just happened.

I want to tell about Mollie because I suspect that somewhere in the telling I'll figure out how it relates to Frank's passage about struggles, not fights. Now, I know there is nothing, absolutely *nothing,* as annoying and cloying as cat lovers simpering over their felines' cosmic virtues. Just last month, a group of us at some local watering hole were nattering about which mythic deities our respective felines were living out in their eighth lives. After fifteen minutes of this, an obviously fed-up graduate student resignedly pushed back his chair, apologized for leaving early, and added, "This is all the kitty support group I can take in one sitting."

Mollie started out as our neighbor's cat. Along with her twin sister Lucy and five other felines of questionable origin, she occupied a house catty-corner from our place. Poor Mollie sealed her fate early on by hissing at her sister and pissing on an oriental rug. "Immature, abrasive, and lacking in good judgment" might well have been the verdict. So Mollie was cast out, where she soon became the neighborhood cat, stealing bits of food and snippets of affection wherever she could find them. She did pretty well for some time. "She's a *very* good hunter," her former owner once rationalized her ousting to me. One day Mollie spotted me on my way to the mailbox. I wasn't particularly impressed with Mollie. She was small, tree-bark gray, skittery, and unfriendly. Her front end was short-haired and silvery, signaling a Russian blue in her lineage somewhere, while her back end was longer-haired and spiked straight up when she stretched, implying a "punk" cat in her background. She had a gray-and-black ringed tail, suggesting that another of her kin might have been a raccoon. More for the hell of it than anything else, I sat down in our driveway and tried my best to mean it when I chirped "Kitty, kitty, kitty." Mollie sauntered over, brushed up against me, and then went unashamedly upside down against the side of my leg. Right there, in that one magical moment, I was hooked.

That was three years ago. From that chance meeting, Mollie has come to own our house. On a night of too many wines and too much purring, I might even have signed my stock portfolio over to her! When I must take her to the vet for her annual shots, I experience my cancer treatment all over again. I mean, is this sick or what? Like it or not, Mollie has become our feline love child.

I got an inkling there was more to it one night when Janice and I were watching television with Mollie, as usual, upside down between us. I was gently rubbing her tummy when Janice looked over, smiled warmly, and said,

"She brings out your softest side. I don't see that degree of tenderness in you very often, and I so like it."

"You do?"

"I do. I really do."

Now *that's* surely news for postmodern man. Women to whom I was attracted in the past did not love my soft side. They always found it weak and unmasculine—something to vilify, not validate. How did my wolfish father put it? "Every time you go ga-ga over some bitch, you just give her your pants and she loses all respect for you. When are you ever going to learn not to spit the bit?" Just hearing Janice's other voice realigned all those old hurts. But what clicked in that moment with Janice was that Mollie represented some fundamental part of me that needs constant attention.

At the time, I didn't think much about what that might be, but an event that happened several months later got me pondering it again. That evening Janice raced into the living room crying "Callie's chasing Mollie!" Callie's a young Airedale whose owners just moved in down the street. In fact, Mr. Callie had introduced us to Callie only a couple of nights before. I remember saying how appreciative I was that he had Callie on a leash. So, where was the leash now? I dashed outside just in time to see Mollie scramble under the fence to our backyard with Callie nipping at her heels, her little body just one bite away from carnage. Some parental protection door in me burst open and I went completely berserk. I snatched up a broken tree branch and gave a very startled young Airedale a serious whack across her butt that she'll not soon forget. Callie bolted up our driveway, heading for home. With stick in hand, I was right on her tail. She darted into her owner's garage, but I was just getting warmed up.

Dripping with sweat, barefoot, panting, and with the stick still firmly clenched in my fist, I stormed up to their front door and punched the bell. Moments later a slightly stunned-looking woman peeked out. I decided to forgo the formalities. "Listen godammit! There's a fucking leash law in this city and you need to start obeying it! Because if that worthless piece of canine shit ever—do you hear me?—*ever!*—comes into my yard again and hurts or kills my cat, you will see Old Testament justice in action. You got that, darlin'?" Me, the anti-Christ of Welcome Wagons. The woman just stood there, dumbfounded. Given my own out-of-control rage, this was, in retrospect, her best option.

So that was the other part of Mollie for me. At that moment, it didn't matter that Mollie never stayed in our yard, or that the leash law I was so self-righteously upholding applied to cats as well as dogs. All that mattered was that Mollie had been threatened, and that I was prepared to defend her to the death. What was there about this animal that I must nurture and protect so passionately? This was a no-brainer. I, the ragingly protective parent, am prepared to defend my feline child against all danger. Ted would have done it for me. I'm sure of that.

On a chill January day I parted company with my two very favorite lymph nodes, and I wouldn't get the pathology report until the next day. In the wee hours I was lying on my back next to Janice, staring blankly. I felt no pain or discomfort but was far too stressed to sleep. I was learning that cancer demons, especially imagined ones, are always bigger and darker and more threatening at night. I lay still because Janice is a very light sleeper. I felt the bed jiggle ever so slightly and smiled because it could only mean that Mollie had joined us and would soon, as she did every night, be snuggling close to Janice. Although we never make a big deal of it, we both know that Janice is the alpha human here. I'm fairly cool in the Molliebolt's eyes, but if there's ever a choice to be made between Janice and me, it's not really a choice.

But tonight something unexpected happened. Mollie began walking up toward Janice's shoulder, her nightly resting place. Then I felt her pause. She seemed slightly agitated, undecided about something. I became aware of the dim outline of her tail twitching. Then she turned, climbed off Janice, came over to me, sniffed lightly near my incision, and bedded down, resting her head softly on top of my dressing. And there she slept, never moving, the entire night. I dropped off soon afterward, but not before feeling an incredible flood of emotion.

I suppose that, on one level, this is no mystery. It took me awhile, but I eventually connected Mollie's laying her head on my wound to my cancer (which, at that time, I didn't know I had). Mollie was showing me a new way of living after cancer. That life form didn't have a coherent structure yet but I was more than ready for it to take shape. I'm fully aware that my long-time therapist, Anne, would throw back her head and howl if someone said they intended to model the rest of their life after a cat. Of course I won't do that. After all, I can't lick my private parts and there's no way in hell I could ever catch a blue-tailed skink!

What I can do is try to understand how Mollie seems to vacillate between intense love and extreme independence without ever losing her unique identity. In many ways, she lives her life, in Frank's terms, more as a struggle and less as a fight. Her kittenish dependence and her hunterish autonomy both seem grounded in a larger individuality. Perhaps her lesson for me is that I too have a larger sense of self within which my various professional voices coexist. If that's true, then one way out of my stuckness is to articulate what that larger sense of myself might be. I believe that's why Mollie came into my life when she did.

Before I could sort this out I got another gift, when I least expected it. No one takes his or her dreams more seriously than Janice. When she can remember them she writes them down, pores over them, and often shares them with me. So, when she recently began one of our breakfasts with "I had a dream," I knew from experience I should listen, even if it wasn't going to be the rhetorical event of the century.

"Oh yeah? What about?" I ask, feigning interest.

"Melting boundaries and unconditional acceptance."

"Is that all?"

"That's all."

"OK, so what do you remember?"

She takes out a 4 x 6 note card, all scribbled over.

"Let's see, I was at school. Yeah, that's right. But this was not another of my 'unprepared for class' school dreams. After ten thousand reruns, I *know* what they mean. This one was different. I was in class and really excited about the material. But I was getting increasingly frustrated because the students didn't share my enthusiasm. The harder I pushed, the more they withdrew. I could feel myself becoming increasingly upset. But then something inside me just sort of snapped, colors changed, and lines distinguishing us began to blur. At one point, it was like a part of me floated above the lectern and began, not so much to look down on the students, although I clearly was at that point, but to see all of us in a larger context. Then a voice in my head began saying over and over, 'We're all doing the very best we can. We're all doing the very best we can.' I felt a great calm pass over me."

She uttered that last line as if it were the conclusion of a sermon. I'm usually pretty facile at sorting out her dreams, but I didn't have the foggiest idea about this one, probably because my own authority issues were rumbling around in there somewhere.

"So, what do you make of it?" she finally asked, when it became clear that I wasn't going to volunteer anything.

"That you've been reading too many Great Goddess books," I delayed.

"No, seriously. I think this one's important, but I just can't get a handle on it."

It was time for me to come up with something.

"Well, I suppose your rising above the group could mean that you're separating yourself out. Maybe it signifies a new and larger space from which to relate to them."

Even as I said these words I saw immediately how applicable that would be for me, so I pushed on. "And I guess that mantra-like 'We're all doing the very best we can' line could imply that, if everyone is already doing the best they can, maybe you could expend less energy on what they might do better, and more on who you might become."

"Now *that* sounds like good advice for both of us."

Collapsing oppositions so that academic life is not always a me-versus-them ordeal; developing a larger sense of self so that I don't always have to play one animal role; envisioning my department as one part of a larger institution instead of some island off by itself; that's a lot to process. As I mulled it over, I remembered an early event, from before my career had taken so many hits. At the time I acted in accordance with those three principals without even knowing it.

One evening I got a call from an ex-student. After making small talk and playing catch-up, he said, "By the way, our department is about to search for a new chair. I've chatted informally with some of my colleagues here, and I—or we—would like you to apply. We think you'd be a very strong candidate. So, what do you think?" I was publishing a lot, teaching large numbers of students, and serving on several important national committees. True, I wasn't all that warm and fuzzy with my colleagues, but we were pretty civil with each other. Acting on impulse mixed with a little hubris, I took a leap of faith: "Oh, what the hell. Why not? What do you need?"

I sent off what he needed, and promptly forgot the whole thing. Imagine my surprise when, several months later, I got a call from the search committee chair.

"Dr. Frentz," she begins, "I'm delighted to tell you that you're one of our three finalists for the chair in the department of Communication. In fact, you're our top-rated candidate."

I am almost as stunned by this news as I was a year earlier when Dr. Logan told me I had cancer. My feelings, however, were quite different.

"*Really?*"

"Really. We'd like to schedule an on-campus interview, but first I need your permission for something."

"Oh, and what might that be?"

"Well, our Dean would like to call the departments of each of our three finalists, just to see how they feel about your potential to be a chair. Would that be all right with you?"

No, it wouldn't. I couldn't imagine anyone saying anything very positive about me. Of course, I couldn't tell her that.

"Well, as long as your Dean doesn't call my parole officer, I guess it would be OK."

"Fine. I'll be back to you in less than a week to set up your interview."

I never expected to hear from her again. I did, however, hear from someone a week later. It was my ex-student, not the search committee chair. No chitchat this time. He got right to the point.

"Geez, Frentz, you must have some real enemies in your department."

"Oh?" I answer, more innocently than I feel.

"I'm sorry to have to tell you this, but our Dean called one of your colleagues, someone he presumably knew, and this guy just trashed you. It was apparently so brutal that the Dean not only removed your name from any further consideration but also refused to listen to our pleas to get some other opinions."

"Can you tell me who this person was?"

"Sure," he says, giving me the colleague's name.

I was surprised, but not all that much. The colleague in question was one of the long-standing, behind-the-scenes movers in the department, a person with a very keen set of political instincts. If this guy were so politically astute, I wondered, why wouldn't he give me an over-the-top recommendation and be rid of me? I was pretty certain it wasn't ethical integrity, but something much more pragmatic. Then it became clear. I was, after all, a productive scholar who taught large numbers of student credit hours for the department. If I were to leave, others might have to pick up the slack. Moreover, being the lowest-paid professor of my rank in the department, I was highly cost effective. Looked at that way, I was neither a problem nor an expense for the department. His hatchet job began to make sense.

I knew that I had to confront my colleague somehow, but the "somehow" wasn't clear. I called my former brother-in-law, Bill Wilmot—a full professor of Communication, nationally acclaimed conflict mediator, and the only Buddhist elk hunter in captivity. I badly needed a crash course in mediation skills. After I told him the gist of what happened, Bill got to the formidable task at hand.

"Get a pencil and some paper."

"Got it."

"All right. Start by making a formal appointment to see him. When you go into his office, close the door. That'll tell him that something serious is about to come down. Now underline this next part. Your objective here is *not* to attack him. Got that? That may well be your instinct, but that's not your goal. If you lose it and fly off at him, he will feel perfectly justified in whatever ugly things he said to the Dean. Your goal is to ensure that he doesn't do this again, should you have another opportunity to be chair. The only way to do that is to be straight and serious without ever attacking him personally. If you're mature in a context where he'll expect you to be just the opposite, then he may question what he said, and, more to the point, he might not say it again. Can you do that?"

"I can try."

"You can do more than try. It's about time you mastered some of the more mature ways to do conflict."

I wrestled with Bill's advice for days. I knew he was right. He was a master at engineering productive conflicts but, given this situation, I recoiled from anything *productive*. It was all I could do to keep from acting out my rage. Eventually, however, I bracketed those baser instincts and began working on a more reasonable game plan. I rehearsed a few scenarios, jotted down some "mature" phrases, and even practiced a few mini-speeches out loud to see how they sounded. I felt like an actor obsessed by learning his lines.

The day finally arrives. Punctual to a fault on that bright Wednesday morning, I walk into my colleague's office, closing the door behind me. He gets up, comes around his desk, and sits in a chair opposite me. Just perfect, I think. Remove any barriers between him and me. Probably something right out of our basic communication skills textbook. Obviously, I didn't quite have the proper attitude yet.

"So, what's up?" he asks cheerily.

"I need to clarify something with you," I answer seriously.

"Oh?"

"A couple of months ago I applied for a chair position. I didn't tell anyone here about it because, well, quite frankly, there wasn't anything to tell. In many ways, I was just testing the water, trying to see if I were marketable. Then several weeks ago, the search committee chair called and said that I was their top choice, and that they wanted me to come in for an interview. Before finalizing the interview, she asked whether their Dean could call someone here about my potential as a chairperson."

My colleague stiffens visibly. I can almost see the wheels spinning in his head, wondering how on earth I knew about a private telephone conversation he had a month ago.

"Having no reason not to, I gave her my permission. Now I've learned that the Dean called you, and that you said some pretty disparaging things about me."

He glances up at the ceiling, obviously stalling—hoping, I presume, for divine guidance.

"Ummm . . . yes . . . that's right," he finally admits. "He did call me."

Nothing from me, but I'm *totally* focused.

"But . . . well . . . ummm . . . you know . . . I can't remember exactly what I said, but I don't think it was anything all that negative. I guess I did mention that you and I had some philosophical differences in the past, but nothing more serious than that," he lies.

"What you said is not important, and it is between you and the Dean," I say. "But whatever it was, it was bad enough that the Dean immediately withdrew my name from consideration. If things had been allowed to run their course, I don't know whether I would have gotten the offer or not. Even if I had, I don't know whether I would have taken it. But I sure would like to have had the choice. Can you understand that? As you know, opportunities for advancement around here are few and far between, and I just had one taken away from me. I'm really hurt and pissed about that."

"I'm really sorry," he says, flushing. "The Dean's call caught me off guard, and I probably spoke out impulsively without really thinking. Would you like me to call him back?"

"No, I wouldn't. The damage has already been done. What I would like you to do instead is to promise me that, should this situation ever arise again, you would at least not sabotage me behind my back. I'm not asking you to lie on my behalf, but I am asking you to treat me with a bit more professional respect. Do you think you could do that?"

"I'd be happy to."

"Thanks."

And with that, I get up, shake his hand, and walk out.

When I told Bill Wilmot what happened, he was thrilled. In this singular episode, I acted in accordance with ideas I would not consciously discover for many years to come. Perhaps this aborted chair opportunity was a prelude to better things, sort of a trial run towards relational maturity.

There it was, an extended episode in which I diminished opposition, acted out of a larger sense of self in an expanded context. Big deal—instead of feeling satisfied and empowered, all I felt was phony and hypocritical. As I relive our conversation now, I still don't believe anything he said, except perhaps the bit about being caught off guard and acting impulsively. Impulses, I've come to learn, often harbor true feelings. What I couldn't figure out was why I so resented acting maturely. Obviously, I could do it if I wanted. What *was* my problem? Recently I got a clue.

I woke from an intense dream that I couldn't remember, sat up in bed, and "heard" two crystal-clear pronouncements. The first: "It's a manhood problem." Yes, of course it's a manhood problem! This whole damned chapter has been about a manhood problem, and I never saw it. I'm in my sixties now. Radiation and chemotherapy may have killed my cancer but they have taken a toll on other areas of my body. I recently developed some "radiation scarring" in my left hip that has caused chronic arthritis. Even as I was writing this chapter, I've been trying to adjust to my first set of hearing aids. When I feel my masculinity declining, as I do now, I turn to the two animals that seem to arrest the feeling, if only for a moment, and that would be my wolf and my coyote. But there are no wolves or coyotes in this chapter. At best, I see only their domesticated offspring, the dog, and dogs don't suggest manliness to me.

Last night I heard a second voice. This one said, "The cruelest cut is to be castrated by eunuchs." That is the source of the repressed rage that runs through this chapter. No matter what kind of spin I put on these episodes, I *feel* that I've been had by weak, sniveling, ineffectual authorities whose own lack of manhood is disguised by their surrogate balls—those rules of structure they use to emasculate me. And, when overcome by those feelings, I revert swiftly and with a vengeance to the extreme form of me-versus-them. Obviously, I still have some work to do with departmental structures and professional colleagues. That work will demand, I now know, more than a book, a cat, and a dream. It's time to revisit my cancer. If clues to the mystery of my manhood and to a better professional life are buried somewhere in my cancer experiences, perhaps it's time to start digging again.

CHAPTER 12

Eye of the Storm

Illness is the experience of living through the disease.

Arthur W. Frank

At the Will of the Body: Reflections on
Illness

I stand next to Thad, sporting my newly installed bio-port and looking at my own x-ray.

"See there?" Thad points to a thin gray line. "That's the catheter tube, right where it should be."

I'm a little too shaky to be impressed.

"Yeah, well, what's that dark mass just to the left?"

"That would be your heart," he answers, as if even Mollie would know that.

"I always figured it would be black," I grumble.

"Well, there it is, empirical evidence of your inherent evil."

"Now what?"

"Now you go down the hall for some nice chemotherapy."

"Will it work?"

"Will what work?"

"The chemo?"

"I told you it would."

"You sure?"

"Yep."

I clutch at that quasi-commitment, grab Janice's hand, and trudge down the hall. The chemo room does not lift my spirits. Like worker bees, nurses and lab technicians come and go from a service island, picking up chemo sacs, IV units, and other related items. Twenty-five Barcaloungers, the kind that tilt all the way back, line the perimeter of the room. Most are filled with patients whose faces register varying degrees of suffering. Where to sit? Anywhere but here, I'm thinking—but here is where I am. We have just about settled on a shop-worn, lime green beauty way off to the side when I hear "Mr. Frentz?" I turn to see a short woman with sharp eyes and auburn hair cut in a Dorothy Hamill.

"Hi," she says cheerily, "my name's Pat and I'll be administering your treatment this afternoon."

"Can I sit over there?" I ask, pointing to the lime green number.

"That'll work."

Pat brings Janice a chair, and even before she sits down I once again latch onto her hand.

"First time?" says an older woman sitting to my right.

"I'm afraid it is," I say tensely.

"Can't even remember my first time anymore," she volunteers. "If my doctors had been right, I'd have been dead four years ago. Cancer all through me, they said. Not much hope and even less time, they told me. But they were wrong, weren't they?" she adds, with a flash of defiance.

"I get hooked up all the time now—guess it keeps the cancer under control. I've plumb wore out five catheters," she says proudly. "I'm such a regular here that they'll probably make me an honorary nurse," she chuckles.

She seems older than I first thought, probably somewhere in her early to mid seventies. She has very thin, mouse-brown hair. With all the chemo she's had, it's a wonder she has any hair at all. Her face is ruddy and round and her smile reveals a questionable set of teeth. She resembles the tough-minded, hard-working German farm women of my childhood. I bet she has a tough skin but a tender soul. She's staring at me.

"So . . . ummm . . . are you all right now?"

Shooting me an if-I-were-all-right-now-would-I-be-here look, she opts for something gentler.

"Well, as 'all right' as you can be at age 52 with terminal cancer."

Fifty-two! The cancer and chemo have definitely taken their toll. She notices, but does not comment on, my extremely insensitive look. Instead, she gives me a simple lesson in living.

"We're all terminal, aren't we? I am feeling better these days. The nausea's an old friend by now, and my hair thins but never does fall out. You hang in there, sonny, you'll come out of this all right. I know some things."

"Yes, you do." I'm fervently hoping she's right. Before I can start to worry about how I'll look when this is over, Pat comes back.

"I'm going to run an anti-nausea drug through your catheter, and then we'll get started." She wheels up a stand with a small sac of colorless liquid suspended from a metal hook, attaches the feeder line to my catheter, turns the petcock, and the puke-no-more starts to flow. I close my eyes and tighten my grip on Janice's hand. Her other hand covers mine tightly. I remain still as I try to breathe evenly.

In no time I hear Pat say, "All right, you're primed and ready. We start with your one-time-only treatment of Mitomycin C." I know all about Mitomycin C, my treatment version of a Molotov cocktail—not as brutal as the potassium-based chemos where you upchuck almost immediately and all your hair falls out in exactly 13 days—but serious stuff nonetheless. Thad had given me a capsule description to read:

> This chemotherapeutic drug is an anti-tumor antibiotic. It inhibits the formation of DNA in fast-growing cells. When mixed, it has a deep blue color, and it is administered directly into the vein in drip form. This takes approximately 30 minutes. Listed below are some of the side effects you may experience while taking this medicine:
>
> • Bone marrow depression
>
> • Mild hair loss
>
> • Nausea and vomiting
>
> • Fatigue
>
> • Loss of appetite
>
> • Irritation at the site of injection
>
> (This drug is very irritating to skin tissues. Report any pain you may feel during administration, or soreness or swelling at the site of treatment.)
>
> • Mouth sores
>
> • Diarrhea

Not exactly a recreational drug.

Pat returns from the island carrying a small pouch of dark blue liquid. She removes the anti-nausea sac and replaces it with the Mitomycin C. I watch as the thick goo oozes its way down the feeder line toward my chest. Suddenly a question pops into my agitated mind: How is this different from what a condemned prisoner experiences in the final moments before a lethal injection? I mean, left to its own devices, this stuff *is* a lethal injection. The only real difference is intent. Politics be damned, this feels like cruel and unusual punishment!

I suck in my chest, unconsciously trying to delay the blue gel's invasion. Mesmerized, I stare as the chemo slowly makes its way down the line. Closer, closer. The entire line is a deep blue now. I wait for any twinge of discomfort. I'm ready—no, I'm *more* than ready—to scream bloody murder at the first sign of pain. None comes. Only a very slight, almost imperceptible, burning sensation at the point of entry. Certainly nothing to scream about. I close my eyes, mentally re-design Green Bay Packer uniforms (my way of passing bad time), and wait.

"There. That wasn't so bad, was it? One down, one to go." My eyes snap open. "The bad one's behind you. Now let's get your pump rigged up, hook you up to the decaffeinated version, and send you home."

Before I can say anything, she's off to Treasure Island again, then back carrying an oversized butt pack, a dispenser pump that looks like a timer for a nuclear device in a James Bond movie, and another sac of clear liquid.

As she programs the pump to shoot 5 cc of chemo into me every twelve minutes for the next ninety-six hours, I think about the decaf. It's fluorouracil, better known in the chemo business as 5FU. It is an old chemo now, but it was experimental back in 1959 when it did absolutely nothing for my mother. To avoid worrying about history repeating itself, I flash back on the handout Thad gave me:

This chemotherapeutic drug interferes with the synthesis of DNA in rapidly growing cells. It accomplishes this purpose by acting on the DNA in three different ways. It is administered directly into the vein and takes approximately 5 to 10 minutes to give.

Listed below are some of the side effects you may experience while taking this medicine:

- Mild nausea and vomiting

- Depressed bone marrow
- Sore mouth
- Diarrhea
- Hair loss
- Fatigue
- Hyper pigmentation of the skin

(This is a darkening of the skin over the vein it was injected into. As treatment continues, this darkening will worsen and follow the line of the vein up your arm. This will resolve after treatment, but may last several months. It in no way affects the condition of your vein.)

A "sore mouth" replaces "mouth sores." And only mild vomiting, as opposed to the richer, more full-bodied kind provided by the Mitomycyn C. But what *are* those three ways 5FU accomplishes its purpose?

As Pat fusses with my chemo camping gear, I glance to my left. I see a strapping young man get unsteadily to his feet. He must be 6'3", about 220 pounds, built like an Adonis, and no more than 20 years old. He's wearing a rumpled white t-shirt, tight faded jeans, and a gold-and-red Kansas City Chiefs cap. I watch as he makes his way slowly, unsteadily, around the island and toward the door. No one seems to notice. Then, almost at the door, he stops, sways slightly, and leans heavily against the wall. His shoulders heave and I hear muffled sobs. First one, then another, of the medical staff embrace him, whispering encouragement. As one holds him, he takes off his hat, bends down, and rests his bald head on her shoulder. After several minutes, he straightens up, puts his cap back on, takes a few deep breaths, and walks out.

I glance at Pat, who answers before I can ask, "It's his last treatment." His last treatment. What an agonizing ambiguity. At this moment, I'm way too frightened to ask. Is he going home to live or die? I never see him again.

In the wizened old woman and the emotional young man I am privileged to see two living examples of people struggling with cancer. Coupled with Arthur Frank's insights, they provided a model for how to *struggle with the illness* as opposed to fighting against the disease.

In memory, my treatment wasn't all that terrible. On the positive side, I never threw up and I usually slept pretty well. I did lose my appetite and my hair thinned and changed texture, but in retrospect those don't seem too bad. Still, I wasn't really prepared for the cumulative effects of radiation and chemotherapy. Several weeks after treatment ended—my bio-port had been removed and placed under my pillow in hopes that the chemo fairy would leave me a treat—I felt worse, not better. That triggered my deepest fears that the treatment had not worked and I was beginning the long, hard ride to the Last Roundup.

When treatment began, I took to sleeping alone in a twin bed on the main floor so as not to disturb Janice, a notoriously light sleeper. I kept my Teddyborg (my chemo back pack) at my side. Strangely, the periodic buzz it emitted when dispensing chemo was a comforting regularity that actually helped me sleep.

One night, slightly more than halfway through the ordeal, things spiraled downward. By this time I had lost my appetite and that, coupled with the intensifying effects of treatment, left me weak and vulnerable. Then too, my two waste disposal systems, usually cooperative and independent, had begun to merge in unpleasant ways, such that when one went off the other did too. So, on this particular evening, I knew better than to reach for a beer.

I tried all my usual tricks, but sleep wouldn't come. I re-designed Packer uniforms, tossed and turned, managing only to tangle up my Teddyborg line, and even recited my chemo mantra, "Let the warm, clear liquid melt away the cold hard cancer," but this just heightened my distress. I even thought of going upstairs, waking Janice and Mollie, and basking in their comfort, but that would have been selfish, and on this night not even they could have helped.

Finally, at 2:47 A.M., wired and tired, I got up and moved to the couch in our study. I half-lay, half-sat, so that I could look out the glass door into the dark April night. As I watched, a spring storm began to develop. At first, I heard small gusts of wind in the oak trees and glimpsed heat lightening far in the distance. Everything intensified as the storm moved closer. The intermittent gusts turned into blasts, and the heat lightening exploded into brilliant chains that flashed, vertically at first, and then, as the storm came upon me, almost horizontal. I sat up, forgetting my discomfort, and lost myself in the beautiful and terrible forces being unleashed. The frequent lightening revealed low-hanging clouds framed by the wildly flaying oak branches.

Then, in the midst of all this summer violence, I turned calm—as if somehow I had magically entered the eye of the storm. I lay back down, closed my eyes, and, just before sleep came, saw in my mind's eye this similar moment in Arthur Frank's book:

Although I never discovered a formula for dealing with pain, I did manage to break through its incoherence one night before it abated. Making my way upstairs, I was stopped on the landing by the sight—the vision really—of a window. Outside the window I saw a tree, and the streetlight just beyond was casting the tree's reflection on the frosted glass. Here suddenly was beauty, found in the middle of a night that seemed to be only darkness and pain. Where we see the face of beauty, we are in our proper place, and all becomes coherent. (33)

This was my face of beauty, my proper place, my moment of coherence. In the eye of that summer storm I came upon my own center, from which I could hope to live differently and, perhaps, better than before.

From that still point, I see things I had never seen. That center is the larger container in which all my various personae and voices reside. If I can stay in the eye of my own storm, I may be able to monitor those voices more carefully and, over time, develop new ones that speak more effectively to my colleagues. In this regard, staying alive means much more than *not dying of cancer*. It also means staying alive psychologically by being more than coyotes, sheep, wolves, or even shepherds. I don't want to abandon my critters—they're too much a part of me for that—but, as John Rodden said earlier, they are not all of me. By staying centered in the eye of my own storm, perhaps I can move beyond them.

It has been well over a year since I was unplugged in the more literal sense of the word. So far, the physical form of staying alive is going well. Like a good vampire, Thad draws and analyzes my blood every three months. Like a good surgeon, Gareth carves a few chunks out of my butt every six months. Like a good patient, I remain cautiously optimistic. On my better days, I think I'm cured, but on my best days, when I feel from my heart, I know better. I am only now coming to terms with the truth about cancer, of which Arthur Frank speaks:

Cancer never disappears. I read recently about a young man whose cancer recurred after a thirteen-year remission. Medical science is just beginning to understand cancer's capacity to be present in the body but inactive for decades. Cancer creates the disturbing image of the body as a time bomb, genetically programmed to explode at some future time. I could be having a recurrence now and not yet know it, or I could live another forty years and die of something else. You are never cured of cancer; you can only live in remission. (130)

Living in remission is the final frontier, the last piece in the puzzle. To live in remission means to stay vigilant, and staying vigilant, for me, means to hunker down in the storm. Just as my body is in remission from cancer, my psyche is in remission from its more destructive impulses, and I must stay alert on both fronts.

Lest I wax too romantic here, it's not always fun to live in (as Frank puts it) "the remission culture." Being watchful over my body forces me to hear, and fear, whatever it might be trying to tell me. A slight twinge here, a quiet pull there, and all the mortality fears flash back in less than a heartbeat. I now get spooked whenever I'm away from my physicians too long. I need more contact with them than I ever did before. I need everybody to stay vigilant. They say they'll keep checking me periodically for five years. After that, they figure, I will have stayed alive. Before I became ill, Janice used to formulate five-year plans for personal, professional, and spiritual growth. I used to groan at those plans; I don't anymore. Her time frame seems just about right.

Most of my animal voices are in remission—at least the more malignant, wolfish ones. Because of that, I have experienced some academic successes of late. We now have a new chair, and when I asked him to support reconfiguring my earlier sabbatical to a medical leave, thus allowing me a legitimate sabbatical to work on this book, he enthusiastically agreed. Last fall, after studying the salaries of all the full professors, I requested a fairly substantial raise. Not only did he support me, but he secured the support of the associate dean as well. Most recently, I asked him to reduce my teaching load to two classes a semester (the normal load being three and two). After listening carefully to my arguments, he said, "Sounds good to me."

From my newfound center, I struggle to stay alert to mind and body. After more than a half-century of living outside that center, old habits die hard. I still flash out impulsively at what I take to be dehumanizing acts, and I will probably always be way too sensitive to minute bodily changes. I would like to end this chapter with the words my favorite author, Robert Pirsig, chose to end his book: "We *have* won it. Things *are* better. You can sort of tell these things" (380). But to borrow Pirsig's ending would be to slip out of the center I have so recently found and regress into my old ways of letting someone else speak for me. I want to speak for myself here. Besides, to "have won it" implies a fight, and I'm more into struggles these days. From the eye of the storm, I can see better. I *can* sort of tell that.

CHAPTER 13

On Becoming a Better Outlaw

And half of gettin' there is knowin' where I been before.

Guy Clark

"Anyhow, I Love You"

I'm up later than usual, re-reading for the umpteenth time Carolyn Ellis' careful commentary on the first draft of this book. I think she's dead center on most everything, but one suggestion keeps hanging me up:

> Yes, I think it is a little short. . . . I'm not suggesting adding a lot. If you tie into literatures here and there and add a chapter maybe, then that would probably do it. I don't know what [a] last chapter would look like. It might be just a scene showing the new Tom, who is still a trickster, for whom life is still an issue but sometimes he makes different decisions than he used to, thinks in different way[s], feels more complexly (if you do). I guess I don't want the new Tom to be presented as perfect—that would defeat the purpose. I guess if it were mine, I'd want to show myself in some context, maybe screwing up a bit, still giving in to my trickster impulses, but then getting out of it by getting to a "loftier" plane or something.

Well damn it, I thought, demonstrating my new maturity. The last chapter *was* the last chapter. It's poignant, holistic, forward-looking, and tied to Pirsig—real literature, for crissake. What more does she want? Do I have to go back into that storm just to anchor this tale with a few more water-logged snippets of life?

Such were my open, receptive, and productive reactions to Carolyn's gentle suggestion that, in its present form, my story didn't feel quite finished. Like most of my infantile tantrums, this one passed, and when it did the grumpy old storyteller got his bearings, sucked it up, and took another hard look at Chapter 12. Carolyn was right. (I just hate it when that happens.) "Let new voices spring from my larger cosmic center." In the cold light of another day, that began to sound like a New Age solution to an age-old problem. I was just singin' in the rain, totally oblivious to *how* I might live better and more fully, only convinced that I *would*.

Then I got the Second Call—not from a cancer specialist or an ex-student, but from a close friend and respected academician at another university.

"What's up?" I ask.

"Our chair just accepted a position elsewhere, along with one of our most productive senior scholars."

"Bummer. Guess they got onto you, huh?"

"We thought we *might* lose both positions—or, at the very least, have them downgraded to assistant professor," he went on, ignoring my jab. "But our dean told us we could maintain both positions, and—here's the good part—at their current senior levels. That means, old buddy, that we now have two full professorships open. How would you and Janice like to apply for them—you for chair, Janice as the senior big deal?"

What on *earth*? Could this be some good karma at last? Is he just leading up to ". . . but first our dean would like to chat with your colleagues?" Or, did this Second Call happen to give me material for my second last chapter?

"Well . . . ummm . . . geez," I stammered. "What an incredible opportunity! Let me run it by Janice and we'll get back to you. Can you cut us some slack? This is all coming pretty fast."

"Oh, sure, this is not a done deal. We're just getting started looking for qualified people, and you two fill the bill. I hope we'll attract a number of strong applicants. From the rumblings I've heard, you and Janice would be very strong candidates. So give it some serious thought, will you?"

"Absolutely."

Janice and I were exhaustive. We consulted our intuitions, made rational lists of pros and cons, and talked confidentially with family and friends. All to no avail. Both of us were hopelessly stuck. If we were fortunate enough to get the offers, our salaries would shoot up significantly. I would be able to conclude my career in a position of power and influence such as I'd never experienced, Janice's reduced teaching load would allow her to concentrate on research projects, and we would be in a place where we were wanted and valued. Still, we would miss our close friends, I would be working 9 to 5, five days a week, 52 weeks a year, and we would leave behind the amenities of a small college town.

Still agonizing over the decision, Janice and I had Jim Beard to dinner. Well-built, wiry, with short-cropped salt-and-pepper hair, Jim resembles the character played by Scott Glenn in *Urban Cowboy*. In the late Sixties and early Seventies, Jim was an organizer for the Vietnam Veterans Against the War. In the mid-Seventies, he moved to the West Coast and joined the Intrepid Trips Information Service of Ken Kesey and the Merry Pranksters, where he wrote manifestos, created acid-trip events, and edited some not-quite-ready-for-prime-time films. Jim eventually returned to this area where, as "Jack Daniels," he became a pioneer in the FM progressive radio movement. In the early Eighties, he made a stab at going straight, rising to vice president of an ad agency.

We met just after Jim bailed out of the ad agency and tripped back into college. As a "non-traditional" student, he wandered into one of my more whacked-out communication classes in the spring of 1986, and that experience—as he usually reminisces after a few Sam Adams—changed his life, although we're not sure it was for the better. He's been my student, my teacher, and a colleague in my current department. At the not-so-tender age of 53, Jim fulfilled his mother's dreams and earned his PhD in Communication Studies from Northwestern University. I sat in on his dissertation defense; he sat in on my cancer defense. Over the years, through good times and bad, he's become the brother I never had, and, because he knows my academic tendencies better than anyone other than Janice, I've come to trust his judgment, so I really wanted to know what he thought when I led off our after-dinner conversation with this not-so-innocent opener.

"I think I've got a pretty good shot at being a chairperson."

"Really?" came his nonplussed response.

"You think I'd make a good chair?" I asked, thinking I would.

"No, I don't."

"Why not?"

"Because your obsessiveness would bury you in the day-to-day details, while you'd get used and abused by wily administrators who would capitalize on your inexperience and exploit your political naiveté, all to the detriment of your department. Once you saw what was going on, you'd go absolutely berserk and send your dean a box of fresh dog shit or something. Then you'd be removed as chair, hated by your faculty for fucking up the department, and marginalized as an outsider. Does that sound vaguely familiar?"

"I think you're working with an old template here," I countered defensively. "I'd be really good with all those reports. I'd have most of them done before they were even requested. Of course I'd be inexperienced in upper echelon political maneuvering and make some mistakes, I know that, but all new chairs have to go through a learning curve, don't you think?"

"No, I still don't think," he said more reflectively. And then this showstopper.

"You're an *outlaw*, man. That's who you are, that's what you do, and that's what you're supposed to do this time around, cancer or no. Chairs, deans, provosts, chancellors—they're all corporate money chasers with PhDs, gotta be or they wouldn't be administrators. That's not you. Real outlaws are few and far between, but they're a priceless lot because they keep some humanity alive in places hell-bent on eliminating it, and when they're as good at it as you are, they birth other outlaws who, in turn, pass those values along to others. That's your calling, always has been. Don't screw it up now by joining the establishment. You ain't as young as you used to be."

I just sat there, letting his words sink in. "You're an outlaw, man." God, that sounded good! But it also sounded dated and dangerous.

"That's old wolf stuff, Jim. Learned it from my dad. Been there, done that, got fired—twice. I hope cancer has taken me beyond that, to a few new ways of living and relating to colleagues," I said, fingering the wolf pendant around my neck.

"Hey, I'm all for growth and change, but if you have to learn some new ways of living, why don't you learn how to become a better outlaw?"

"How to become a better outlaw?" Trickster words for sure. I liked the sound of that too, but didn't trust it any more than I did the rush I felt earlier. Maybe I was thrilled over not having to change. That would make sense. Non-change is always easier than change. But the more I thought about it, the more I came to trust this better-outlaw image. *Outlaw* was clearly a gloss on "trickster." No mystery there. But "better" was the key, because it implied, among other things, a different way of relating than the one I used to practice. "Become a better outlaw." Maybe I could do it, but first there was the chairperson issue to resolve.

I awoke the next morning haunted by Waylon Jennings' song, "Don't You Think This Outlaw Bit's Done Got Out of Hand?" Last night's fantasy about being the Keith Richards of rhetoric had faded and I was recycling to the still-tempting chairperson opportunity.

"So, Janice," I start off. "You realize we might be able to almost double our current salaries if I got offered this chair position and you went as Dr. Senior Scholar."

"You're probably right," she says, not exactly giving a ringing endorsement.

"So, what do you think?" I push. "Worse case scenario is we get two offers, use them to up our salaries here, and then respectfully back away."

"I couldn't do that and neither could you. I know that's the way these things are done, but that's not the way we do them. These people are friends. Remember Jim talking about humane values? 'Use 'em and abuse 'em' doesn't sound all that humane to me," she concludes, with more than a touch of ethical finality.

I sit with that for a minute, knowing she's right, but not wanting to give up too quickly on what may be my last opportunity for promotion. She's not finished.

"Besides," she continues, "we're at a point in our lives where we need to look at the total picture, not just our academic careers. We've been here— what?—seventeen years now. We've made close friends, your son lives close by, we have a wonderful home in a one-of-a-kind location, and we enjoy the relaxed comforts that come from living in a small, quiet college town," she says, ticking off all the advantages we'd discussed before.

"And you know what else?" she says. "We really don't need any more money. We're doing just fine. Make more, spend more, pay more taxes. That's just crazy. Besides, I don't have much enthusiasm for moving again. I can see the benefits, but after what Jim said last night, I have no willingness."

"Me neither," I respond, with a touch of sadness. "But what's the challenge if we stay?"

"Why don't you try to become that better outlaw?"

"Because I don't know how to do that."

"I don't either," she confesses, "but why don't you think about it? My guess is that you've already *been* a better outlaw and if you could remember a few of those incidents you might be able to use them as models for living a higher-quality life."

What would it mean to become a better outlaw? That seemed to be the question. But as I mulled it over I came to see it needed reframing. The real question was how I could honor my colleagues while still challenging some of the structures in which we work. Could I question unjust procedures without threatening people? I remember saying in my wolf voice, "Save the person, savage the structure." Easier said than done. However, if Janice was right that I'd already done this, it might be a good place to start.

I recalled those hostile minutes I used to submit as faculty secretary. Clearly, they represented my worst-outlaw mode, as I attacked people and structures indiscriminately. Then I flashed forward to my current status as secretary of the Rhetoric and Public Address division of a regional organization. Was I still acting up? The minutes of business meetings are about as interesting as hog futures. Could I undermine the structures, but not the people who lived in them?

I discovered there was a learning curve. For a few years, I wrote two sets of minutes. The "persona" minutes were ditch-water dull, but they regularly appeared in the summer newsletter, and were indistinguishable from the reports of the other division secretaries. The "shadow" minutes I sent to a select few in and out of the region who might appreciate my unexpurgated thoughts. They were wildly inappropriate, undisciplined, and so deadly accurate about the players that even I wince today at my careless insensitivity.

Over time, word of these shadow minutes spread throughout the region. I began getting requests for the "real" minutes of the Rhetoric and Public Address meetings. Obviously, I was delighted with the requests, but loath to go public. Then John Lucaites, one of those upon whom I'd inflicted the darker notes, suggested that I just submit them to the newsletter and see what happened. "If that's all you send," he reasoned, "that's all they'll have to print."

So I gave it a try, but changed a few things first. By infusing a personal, ethnographic voice into the usual goings-on, I came up with a hybrid form that was both lively and informative. Much to my surprise, the first set of these minutes not only was accepted but also appeared on the last page of the newsletter. Not long after, I got an email from a longstanding pillar in the division, saying he couldn't wait to read the next set of minutes! Maybe I'd stumbled onto one way of being a better outlaw.

To compare, I retrieved two recent issues and read my remarks. I was drawn to this section from my 2001 minutes:

> Consider, for example, how we selected our VP-elect. Best I can figure, Jon Paulson nominated Mary Stuckey by email, Mary replied by email that if elected she would govern, and because no one had his or her laptop at the meeting, Mary just became our first virtualized VP-elect, sort of by tacit electronic acclamation. And, because I'm not at all sure about her status as an "original," it might be best if we all think of Mary as a second-order simulation in the Baudrillardian sense until or unless her ontic status proves to be otherwise. (28)

I transformed the awful report language of divisional elections into a bizarre fusion of technology, postmodern theory, and outrageousness. Most important, I never seriously questioned the professional reputations of Jon Paulson and Mary Stuckey. Was this an anomaly or was I really onto something? Here's my opening gambit from the 2002 minutes:

Interlude 1
In a rare leisure moment one day, depth psychologist, C. G. Jung thought about relationships that were neither causal nor coincidental. For lack of a better term, he called this relational halfway house *synchronicity* and defined it as a "meaningful coincidence."

Interlude 2
Bill: "Hey man, what's up?"
Me: "The R & PA minutes, that's what's up."
Bill: "Cool. So how you gonna butcher 'em this year?"
Me: "You know, I'm clueless. This séance has me stumped. I just can't get a lock on it. I'd almost rather write about the cat show that was going on across the street from the convention."
Bill: "Bingo, buck-o! There's your analogy for this year."
Me: "You're a very sick person, William, but of course you're right." (35)

These two interludes dramatize how I came up with my rather outlandish analogy, which runs through the minutes, all the while covering the topics all minutes must address. Using humor, I critiqued a part of academic structure by comparing it to a cat show, all the while preserving the reputations of those in the division. At least in this way, I have already been that better outlaw.

But what about my current job? Are there any signs that I have been a better outlaw here? One answer comes to mind.

I've just finished my last Fine Arts Film Lecture, sort of cyberpunk rap on the 1982 science fiction classic, *Blade Runner*. As always happens, fifteen to twenty-five students are hanging around to hear a few more behind-the-scenes stories, and to argue over whether the main character is a replicant (synthetic person) or a human. Although I'm tired after a three-hour class, I never hurry the hangers-on because they are the most involved students. Eventually all drift off, save one. I recognize the face—guys with three silver rings through their right eyebrow are hard to forget—but in a class of 215 I've never met him. As I gather my things, he just stands around.

"Mind if I tag along to your office?"

"Tag along," I say, gearing up for still another "here's-why-I've-got-to-have-a-B " story. But that never materializes.

"So," I begin as we walk, "what's your name?"

"Billy Joe."

"I never trust guys with two first names," I say, shooting him a look that I hope tells him I'm just kidding.

"You can trust me," he shoots back.

"And why is that?"

"Do I *look* like a Billy Joe?"

"You got me there, B.J."

We get to my office, and Billy Joe holds my stuff as I unlock the door. He sits down and begins to case the joint—for clues to my being, I guess.

"I really like your tie-dye T-shirt," he says unexpectedly. "Where'd you get it?"

"A graduate student's dad custom-made it for me several years ago. My son is the percussionist in a New Orleans horn band and I wanted one that would reflect Mardi Gras colors," I say, revealing a bit more than I usually do to guys named Billy Joe.

"I took a history course last fall called something like 'The Culture of the 60s.' It was a pretty cool class. Those hippies really kicked some establishment ass back then. Wish I'd been around. Didn't they wear tie-dyed T-shirts and jeans?"

"A lot of them did."

"Where you a hippie?"

"No, I was more of a wolf," I say before I can catch myself.

"What happened to all those hippies?"

"Most of them turned into sheep and began eating the grass they used to smoke."

He chuckles knowingly, then nods towards my pendant, "Is that a wolf around your neck?"

"Yep."

He leans in. "He doesn't look ferocious enough to be a wolf."

"Well, he's mellowed some over the years," I smile, "but he used to be extremely ferocious."

"Really? How did he manage to stay alive?"

"Now *that*, Billy Joe, is a long story. Tell you what. Kick back, have a great summer, get some metal in your other eyebrow for symmetry, and in the fall, if you're still interested, come back and I'll tell it to you."

"I'll be back," he says with conviction.

"I'll be here, " I say with hope.

So maybe, if I don't teach B.J. how to build a pipe bomb, I can be a better outlaw with students too. But I've always been a better outlaw with students like B.J. My earlier experiences with Jim Beard seem to affirm that. Clearly, I have done this better-outlaw/trickster bit with professional colleagues who I see once a year at conventions and with marginalized students looking for a professorial champion. But the real conundrum, the one I've been trying to finesse, has always been my day-to-day relationships with authority figures. I can dodge all I want, but I'm still mired in that relational dilemma, and I think Carolyn Ellis meant that I could not end this tale until I came to some resolution, even if provisional, to that problem.

Somehow, I felt I had to tough this one out alone. This issue belonged to me, not Janice, not Jim Beard, not anyone else. I was stuck again, and I stayed that way for almost four months, writing a little, stressing a lot. I thought about Bill Wilmot's Buddhist-like advice for transforming conflict. Whenever he was really angry at someone, when all his impulses told him to run and hide, he did just the opposite and approached the person for a talk. I considered that, but couldn't even entertain the idea. Why? Something was holding me back, and I couldn't get a handle on it. So I stayed stressed and stuck. Then, just as Pirsig and Jung had promised, I got a break.

I had been getting up early for almost a month. I would pour a cup of coffee, sit in the living room, and do a quasi-meditational exercise. I liked the routine because it centered me for the day. Then, one morning in August, at the tender age of 64, I felt a sudden anxiety. Without thinking, I broke my routine and walked toward the study where I had spent that long night "in the eye of the storm." At the end of the hall, just outside my study, hangs a knife, box-framed in walnut. As I looked at it, a ray of sun glanced off my computer screen and onto the shiny brass plate below the knife. The inscription reads, "The Randall Knife." Janice had given it to me for my sixtieth birthday, and, when it became obvious that I would never actually cut anything with it, she had it framed for Christmas several years later. Smiling at all the memories this gift contained, I turned back down the hall but I only took four steps before it hit.

"The Randall Knife" is both a knife and the title of a song written by Guy Clark. To understand the knife is to understand the song, and to *really* understand the song, I was about to learn, was to break up the energy that was keeping my colleagues at arm's length. I first heard Guy Clark on a Sunday afternoon in 1977, when a group of close-knit friends, bonded together by the pain of relational failures, was in the process of getting royally smashed. At the time, "The Reamers and Screamers," as we subtly called ourselves, were also into outlaw country music. Someone put this new album on, but we were all too buzzed to pay it much mind. Then a few of us caught a lyric or two, then a few more, and soon no one was making a sound. After the final cut on the first side, there wasn't a dry eye in the room. Maybe it was the line, "Whoever said the hand is quicker than the eye has never tried to brush away a tear." From that moment on, I was hopelessly hooked on Guy Clark and his remarkable story songs of life north of the border.

Clark wrote "The Randall Knife" in 1983. I've listened to it countless times, in concert, on vinyl, on audiotape, and now on CD. I've played it for strangers, friends, and intimate others—and I've never made it through without crying. Here are the lyrics:

My father had a Randall knife.
My mother gave it to him,
When he went off to World War II
To save us all from ruin.
If you've ever held a Randall knife,
Then you know my father well.
If a better blade was ever made,
It was probably forged in Hell.

My father was a good man,
A lawyer by his trade,
And only once did I ever see
Him misuse the blade.
It almost cut his thumb off,
When he took it for a tool.
The knife was made for darker things,
And you could not bend the rule.

He let me take it camping once,
On a Boy Scout jamboree,
And I broke half an inch off
Tryin' to stick it in a tree.
I hid it from him for awhile,
But the knife and he were one.
He put it in his bottom drawer,
Without a hard word one.

There it slept and there it stayed,
For twenty-some odd years.
Sort of like Excalibur,
Except waiting for a tear.

My father died when I was forty,
And I couldn't find a way to cry,
Not because I didn't love him,
Not because he didn't try.

I'd cried for every lesser thing,
whiskey, pain, and beauty.
But he deserved a better tear,
And I was not quite ready.

So we took his ashes out to sea,
And poured 'em off the stern.
And threw the roses in the wake
Of everything we'd learned.
When we got back to the house,
They asked me what I wanted.
Not the law books, not the watch,
I need the thing he's haunted.

My hand burned for the Randall knife,
And there in the bottom drawer,
I found a tear for my father's life,
And all that it stood for.

Now my wife has given me a Randall knife, and perhaps it could, if I ever grasped its import, lead me toward a better life. But, what is its import? What "darker thing" was it made for? Hell, I'm a rhetorical critic and this is a text, I should be able to figure it out. On the surface, the song tells of learning how to appreciate a father's life, and eventually to mourn his death. I thought I buried my father way back there in Chapter 4, so why do I find more tears for his life every time I hear this song? I walked back to my own Randall knife, and just stood before it. Then I heard something like, "You have not yet found what your dad's life stood for, and until you do you won't be able to find a proper tear." So I cranked up my critical instincts and dug in.

It is obvious to even a first-time listener that this is a story about a son's struggle to grieve the death of his father. The mother gives her husband a knife to protect him in war. It is not an ordinary knife, but one hand-forged by W. D. "Bo" Randall. "If you've ever held a Randall knife, then you know my father well," the son tells us. "If a better blade was ever made, it was probably forged in Hell." What might that say about the father? That he has a sharp edge, a dark side, perhaps even a dangerous side.

And then the son says, "My father was a good man, a lawyer by his trade, and only once did I ever see him misuse the blade. It almost cut his thumb off when he mistook it for a tool. But the knife was meant for darker things and you could not bend the rule." In the song, the son moves quickly over the lines, "My father was a good man, a lawyer by his trade." Why? Perhaps because the lawyer is not the father he most loves and respects. This good man, this lawyer by trade, tries to use the knife as a tool, but this knife is meant for darker things. Was this good lawyer also made for darker things? So it would seem. The son takes the knife on a Boy Scout Jamboree and breaks half an inch off trying to stick it in a tree. He dulls the father's edge and then tries to hide it from him, but he cannot because "the knife and he are one."

Could this boy, by breaking the point, have broken his connection to that part of his father that he loves best, the part that's meant for darker things? Is that the part of the father, along with his damaged blade, that is buried in some psychic bottom drawer "without a hard word one"? "There it stays and there it sleeps for twenty-some odd years," the son goes on, "sort of like Excalibur waiting for a tear." A pretty archaic image for a Texas poet: Excalibur, the blade young Arthur must extract from a stone to prove he is the future king of England. What's that mythic image doing in a country song?

Perhaps the son must extract this small sword from the bottom drawer to recover the darker part of the father that has been enshrined there for twenty-some odd years. "When we got back to the house, they asked me what I wanted. Not the law books, not the watch, I need the thing he's haunted. Oh my hand burned for the Randall knife, and there in the bottom drawer, I found a tear for my father's life and all that it stood for." A son's tear for his father's other life, not the "good man," not "the lawyer by his trade," but the life that is one with a knife made for darker things.

What does all this have to do with my father and me? It took Guy Clark twenty years to find a tear for his father's life, but I seem to find tons of tears for my own father's life every time I listen to his song. For some, my father too was a good man, a banker by his trade, but for me and countless others, he was a bad man, a charismatic rogue with a self-destructive set of authority issues. Those who knew him well either loved him or loathed him; there was no in-between with my dad. He made sure of that. My mother mostly loathed him, because he was unfaithful, emotionally absent, and immature. I loved him because he rescued me from my mother and initiated me into the rites of manhood in Wisconsin. I never did connect with the good man, the banker by his trade—only the wolf, that hostile rebel who hung out with convicts and social misfits and did things no self-respecting banker should ever do.

My father died when I was 33, a little over a year after I had gone West like a young man should. I don't know how Guy Clark's father died, but I know that Ted shot himself. Suicide is always an intensely personal decision, and no one can ever know how that decision is made. Did his emphysema progress to the point where he couldn't breathe? Did he miss me more than he ever let on? I'll never know. I do know that, like Guy Clark, I never found a tear for my father's life. But unlike Guy Clark, I knew exactly why. I was still way too angry over that lost decade when I tried to replace my mother in both of our lives.

I may not have found the tear, but I did find something else. I found, rehabilitated and lived out, my father's dark side. No breaking a point off the knife here. No bottom drawer for me. I honed my father's most self-destructive edges to razor sharpness. No mere wolf for this boy; only an alpha wolf would do. Where he only talked about getting fired, I actually got fired—more than once. Where he *almost* got busted for bad-mouthing cops, I really did get busted for bad-mouthing cops—more than once. Looking back, I see I was still furious at him, always trying to one-up him, always trying to do him one better, always saying, in effect, "Here asshole! You want to get fired? Here's how you *really* do it. You want put down cops? Watch *this!*" I was always living for and through him.

Now it comes, the meaning of this haunting song. I do not need to replicate my father's dark side to find the proper tear; I need to bury the blade with him where it belongs. Tom Whitebear once said if ghosts aren't buried properly, they come back to haunt you (Pirsig 31). How do I become a better outlaw or, to put a slightly different spin on it, a compassionate coyote? Stick the blade back into the rock. That's the key to this father complex. If I can do that, I can nurture a trickster-grounded masculinity that still traffics in relational oppositions, but no longer needs to destroy the opposition. I think that's an important difference. Thanks, Guy.

CHAPTER 14

Last Call

Oh, how shall heaven crown that gold-gleamed hair.
Deb Sabo
"For Janice"

We both hear the phone, but Janice picks up the receiver in our kitchen. Her back is to me, the mid-day sun bouncing playfully off her golden hair, but we both feel the tension.

"Hi, Dr. McFadden," she says. "Thanks for getting back to me so quickly."

I am heading for the extension in the study.

"Janice. I have some bad news. You don't have an inner-ear infection. Your MRI showed multiple lesions on your brain. Now I've already scheduled two CT-scans in the morning to see if we can locate the source of these lesions."

"Hi Connie, Tom here. Are lesions tumors?" I hear myself ask.

"They can be, but we're not sure. We think of them as abnormalities."

I can't recall anything else. When I hang up, I already know and I think Janice knows too. My eyes fill with tears as I walk back into the kitchen. Janice is standing near the sliding glass door to our deck, her back still to me. Slowly, I turn her around and look at her cherished face. She looks dazed and frightened.

I hold her tightly until tears stream down both our faces. We know that our lives, after thirty years of being together, are about to change radically, and not for the better.

Several weeks later, in late January, Janice's radiation treatments are almost finished, but the hoped-for improvement, although we knew it would be temporary, has never come. The treatments have drained Janice's energy reserve, and she didn't have all that much to begin with.

She sleeps well. Small blessings. We wake around 6:30 and I head down to bring up coffee. I used to bring two cups, but Janice has been losing her taste for coffee. Now I bring one, and sometimes she's up for a sip or two. Not this morning.

We sit up in bed, propped up with pillows, Mollie cuddled up tightly against Janice's thigh, looking at the sunrise. It's glorious. Thin dark clouds band the horizon and, as the sun comes up, beams of peach and gold streak above the cloud cover. We don't speak. Out of the corner of my eye, I watch Janice closely, trying to fathom what must be going through her mind. She's watching the rising sun when I see her lips move. Almost inaudibly she asks, half to me and half to the sun, "I'm not going to make it, am I?"

I get up, come around the bed, and sit next to her. She doesn't look at me, but continues to stare out the window. I take her hands and see tears well up in her eyes as I do. If only I could lie, give false hope, put on a happy face, but I'm not made that way and so I don't. "No, my love, you aren't going to make it. It's in too many places and has gone too far. All I can promise is to be right here, at your side, helping all I can, trying to feel some of what you feel, and holding you close until you must let go." The tears flow down her cheeks as she looks at me and squeezes my hands.

"What are you feeling, right now?" I ask, not knowing what else to say or do.

"Sometimes . . . sometimes," she says, "I'm actually all right with it, at peace with it. Other times I'm just so frightened."

I hold her now, and feel her arms around my back. I can feel the weakness in her touch, sense the fear within her heart. We just sit there like that for who knows how long. From that morning on, every day is much worse than the one before. No plateaus, no reprieves, no flat periods, no holding patterns—just progressive and rapid decline. Eventually, what I pray for changes.

At her oncologist's urging, we try chemotherapy, not the chemo-lite that I endured, but the platen-laced tough stuff. Thank God, Janice and I don't have to face this alone. Janice's best friend, Gale Young, flies in from California to be with us.

On an early February afternoon we sit in a crowded waiting room of the local chemo shop. My mood is so different from when I had my first chemo treatment four years earlier. Back then I was frightened, to be sure, but also hopeful. I just kept repeating Thad Carlson's mantra, "I can cure this" and clung to the hope that he could. No such hope here. Although I've never told anyone this, a friend confided that the radiologist who read Janice's MRI said he'd never seen a worse brain scan. So why are we doing this?

The wait seems endless, but eventually a nurse emerges from the chemo room and calls Janice's name. The room is similar to the one I entered in 2000, a large rectangle ringed with recliners filled with sick people. Gale and I look at Janice and see that she's too distraught to sit in the main arena. We spot two rooms off to the side, curtained and containing hospital beds. These are apparently reserved for the gravely ill. We commandeer one; Janice surely qualifies. But even then, with some privacy, I have a bad feeling about this.

After a few minutes, a woman yanks back the curtain. She seems none too pleased that we chose this room and not one of the recliners out front. Her nametag reads "Vivian." She takes one look at Janice and clicks into what is presumably her "mother role." "Hi, hon," she says with syrupy sweetness. "This your first treatment?" Janice says nothing. Gale and I say nothing. My bad feeling escalates.

Janice doesn't have a catheter, so Vivian needs to insert an IV. It takes her three tries. As she finally sets the needle, I feel Janice's nails dig into my hand and see tears stream down her cheeks. The bad feeling turns to anger. Granted, Janice has small arms and even tinier veins, but these people are supposed to be experts with IVs—that's what they *do*, for crissake! I flash back to those CT-scan chimps who messed with me three years earlier, and wonder if Vivian learned her craft from them. But I say nothing.

After the anti-nausea fluid, Vivian hooks up the chemo bag and has Janice swallow a couple of pills. Immediately, Gale and I see that something is wrong. Janice becomes very agitated and it takes all Gale and I can do to keep her on the bed. I catch Gale's eye, and we're both terrified. I've had chemo, granted not this industrial-strength stuff, but this should not be happening.

"Vivian, something's really wrong here."

"Well, she does seem pretty upset, doesn't she?"

"Could you please call Dr. Bloom and have him check on her?" I say. No wolf here. I'm too concerned about Janice to even feel like attacking.

"Dr. Bloom isn't in today," Vivian says.

I glance at Gale, and she back at me. How, we both wonder, can an oncologist "not be in" when one of his patients is getting her first chemo treatment?

"Please," I beg, "could you get some oncologist on call to check Janice. This is not a normal reaction."

Reluctantly, Vivian leaves, while Gale and I try our best to calm Janice. Finally, Vivian returns with none other than Malcolm Woodward, the oncologist that Paula steered me away from four years ago. I am about to find out why.

"What seems to be the problem?" he asks with irritating indifference.

"Is this sort of agitation normal for a first chemo treatment?"

Woodward studies Janice for a moment and then says, "Well, she does seem upset." He picks up Janice's chart. After glancing at it quickly, he looks up. "Poor woman. You'll have a feeding tube put in soon, I suspect."

Gale and I just stand there dumbfounded, totally immobilized by fear and ignorance. As I write this I long for my wolf, but at the time he's nowhere to be found. This is sheep territory and we're totally dependent upon this so-called expert.

"OK, give her 25 cc Demerol," he says, and turns to go. They give Janice the Demerol and she falls mercifully asleep for the duration of her treatment. In early evening Gale and I lovingly carry an only semi-conscious Janice to my car and take her home. Only later do we discover that, even though we told Dr. Bloom that Janice was allergic to Ambien, the usual sedative used to calm frightened chemo patients, somehow that message never got through to Vivian. Those two innocent-looking pills she had Janice take before her treatment did the damage.

In retrospect, I think Janice's one chemotherapy treatment accelerated her death—and I'm not sure that was a bad thing. Although she drifted in and out of consciousness for a few days, she soon slipped into a coma from which she never emerged. Gale cancelled her return flight, Janice's sister Joyce, her husband Gary, Janice's brother Ed, and her parents all flew in immediately. I contacted hospice, who equipped Janice with oxygen and an automatic morphine pump. We began our vigil.

It is mid-evening, two weeks later.

"Why don't you get a couple hours sleep?" my friend Joel suggests. "We'll let you know if anything changes."

"I'll try. I could use some rest."

I leave Janice's study, walk past the Randall knife, and head across the hall to our guest room. The oxygen machine drones steadily as I kick off my shoes and crawl under the covers fully clothed. Although I don't expect to, I fall asleep immediately.

"Tom."

It's Joel, and there's some urgency in his tone.

"I think she's going."

More asleep than awake, I grab one shoe and mechanically begin to put it on. Then Joel's words fully register. I stumble to my feet and hobble across the hall, one shoe on, one shoe off. Not a moment too soon.

Joyce is bending over Janice, her cheek pressed tightly to her temple. I gently take her head in my hands, hearing her breath now, uneven, ragged—not the piston-like rhythms of the past few days.

"We're at the boat, my love," I whisper into her ear. "I'm going to let go of your hand now. Just get on. It will be all right. Fine, really. I love you with all my heart. I always have, I always will. You know that. It's time to go. I will always, *always*, be here. Wait for me. Save me a seat, OK?"

Janice's breath shortens, then one long intake, an exhale, then nothing as she stiffens ever so slightly. Numbly, I glance down at my watch. It reads 9:43 P.M. Joyce collapses to the floor and sobs in her mother's lap. I hear Janice's parents crying softly in the dark. Joel and Jean—friends of magnitude beyond words—stand like sentinels as we try to comprehend the incomprehensible. Janice is dead, of cancer, exactly forty-four days after that phone call.

I feel nothing. No, that's not true. I feel relieved, incredibly relieved. With no chance, no hope, I no longer prayed for Janice's life, but rather for her quick and painless death. I guess that prayer was answered.

For almost twenty-three years, I spent virtually twenty-four hours of every day with Janice. That's unusual. Because of that constant contact, our friends, even our very close friends, often misread our relationship. In the argot of the Eighties, they thought we were the poster couple for co-dependency, but they were wrong. Janice and I are both introverts who need solitude and personal space for psychic renewal. And so we developed elaborate patterns of parallel play where we were in each other's presence and also in our own heads.

Perhaps because of that, or because my own grief began with that ominous January phone call, I survived the hours, days, and weeks that followed better than most expected. "How are you doing?" friends would ask. My answers varied. To those closest to me, I gave my most honest response: "Shit-ty." To others, I said "There are bad days, and then there are worse days." And to those who I thought should not have asked (although I understood why they did), I gave a wolfish version of "Well, I've neither eaten my gun nor run off with a 13-year-old cheerleader, so I must be doing all right."

There's no manual for grief. At least if there is, I haven't found it. Like everyone else, I just muddle along, having a few good days and lots of ghastly ones. For me, however, it works best to balance the solitary grief of being here, in our home with her memories and energy, with more public forms that I share with family and friends. Two adventures on the public seas really helped me stay afloat.

Immediately after her death, Janice's family and I decided to hold a memorial service at the university. We hoped it would be a place where colleagues, students, and friends could honor her life and bid her goodbye. I thought I knew how much Janice was valued in her profession, but I was clueless. The room held 375 people, and it was full. People flew in from all over the country, many literally insisting that we allow them to say a few words. What began as a local gesture quickly turned into a national event.

I prepared some remarks, of course. I'd gone over them, anticipating the "hard parts," and tried to prepare myself for what I knew would come. I had a great opening:

> At 4:52 P.M., June 13, 1981, on a glorious Colorado afternoon in the modest sanctuary of Central Christian Church in northern Boulder, Janice and I were married. Many of the usual suspects are back with us again tonight. Rick Frost co-led the service with Janice's father. Jan Frost stood near and held us close. My son Mark sat up front and delivered the rings. Bill Wilmot blessed our union. Vera Potapenko read a poem Tom Farrell had written for the occasion—a poem, incidentally, which still graces the wall of our home. And Joyce Hocker left us with these words: "Kiss the joy as it flies, live in eternity's sunrise, and be kind to each other." We always tried to do that. ("Three" 1)

That was as far as I got. It's hard to cry in front of 375 people. I thought of Joyce's comment, "Tears flush away pent-up emotions." And so I just stood there, as if I had another choice, until the grief subsided. There were other times I had to stop, but each time taught me a valuable lesson. When people share your loss, they welcome your feelings. But in March 2004 those feelings were still pretty raw.

The second memorial service, although it wasn't officially called that, occurred in Chicago at the National Communication Association's national convention. Two back-to-back panels were scheduled, the first to honor Janice's scholarship, the second dedicated to her life. I was on the second one. Truth be told, I was not looking forward to this convention or this panel; it would be the first convention since 1971 that I attended without Janice, and I'd already struggled through one memorial service. I knew, well in advance, that this would be another very difficult time, but a time that I needed to endure—all part of that never-ending healing process.

But what could I possibly say that I hadn't said already? As soon as I asked the question, I knew the answer. Every summer for almost twenty-five years, Janice and I drove to her parent's cabin high on the western slope of the Colorado Rockies, about halfway between Gunnison and Crested Butte. It was our best time—always, without exception. It was the only place where Janice could relax and regenerate. "They can't get at me here," she would say wistfully, referring to the crushing demands that accompany someone who has become a nationally known figure in her field. For obvious reasons, we never owned a cell phone, and saw that as some kind of a moral victory.

This time I would be driving to the cabin alone, and I would take with me, not my beloved Janice, but rather her ashes—to be buried, as she had requested of Joyce many years ago, in the remote and beautiful cemetery in Tincup, Colorado. My remarks at the convention told of that drive, of that summer, and of my continuing struggles to deal with her loss. After the service, after interring Janice's ashes, after most have left, I feel something is still unfinished.

I need to imprint this place. Janice and Joyce found it many years ago, and Joyce told me that Janice said at the time, "I want to be buried here someday." Now is that time. Today is that day. From Janice's gravesite I look across a lush meadow, cut through with fast-flowing streams and inhabited by at least two beaver families, who, I know from experience, will dam the streams and change the water flow in ever-renewing patterns. The meadow embraces every shade of green imaginable, from the lime-yellow hues of new growth through the deep forests of mature grasses, all the way to the orange-greens of dormant stalks. My eyes lift to the foothills, cloaked in the emerald of lodge pole pines and the blue-green of lush spruces. Every so often, I catch sight of an Aspen grove, and know that in less than a month, those will turn a brilliant peach in stark contrast to the verdant conifers. Above the foothills, at timberline, I see Cumberland Pass at 12,000 feet. Bracketing the pass on the right is Green Mountain, and on the left Fitzpatrick Peak, both majestic 13,500 footers still laced with patches of last winter's snow.

I see all of this, and know that Janice does as well. I stand to leave, take a few steps, but then pause, feeling somehow conflicted. Unfinished business. I think about the chorus of the old country song, "Ashes of Love," that I borrowed for the title of this convention paper. It goes:

> Ashes of love,
> Cold as ice.
> You made the debt,
> I'll pay the price.

That chorus may be just right for the song, but it's all wrong for this moment. Try this:

> Ashes of love,
> Still burn in my heart.
> I leave you here now,
> But we're never apart.

There. Much better. Time to head home now. (*"Ashes"* 202-03)

But the tributes to Janice did not end here. After this panel, numerous friends, colleagues, and ex-students approached me and pleaded for some forum in which they too might express their admiration and love for Janice. Art Bochner contacted John Meyer, editor of the *Southern Communication Journal*, and asked whether John would consider a special issue devoted to Janice's life and scholarship. John graciously agreed. Art and I shared the guest editorship and, in the summer of 2006, the issue came out.

"Has anyone within our discipline ever had an entire issue of a scholarly journal devoted to him or her?" someone asked me. I didn't know, and so I asked around. Nobody could remember this ever having been done before. I am only now coming to realize how amazingly fortunate I have been. For almost thirty years I have known, loved, and lived with a woman whose soft, gentle kindness could not hide the charismatic radiance of her voice and her presence. I always knew Janice was special, but I never realized how many other people thought so too. As my colleague said, I was over-rewarded.

The personal grief is harder to manage because it always sneaks up on me when I least expect it. Some things Janice and I used to do together (like shopping) now seem so empty and sad that I no longer do them, while others (like having a few drinks and dinner with students and colleagues) feel all right and I continue them. Sometimes I'll be reading a book and be brought up short by a note Janice wrote in the margins. Other times I'll be wrestling with one of her recipes and freeze at the sight of her handwriting. I get caught off guard by those things, but that's just the way it is right now.

The most difficult things come from within. I am to teach Janice's myth seminar in the spring of 2005, and to reacquaint myself with the material I have been rereading Jung. And that includes the "shadow," that most odious and disowned part of our personality. No big deal, I *know* the shadow. In fact, one of my less savory but more enduring roles has been as the target for lots of people's projected shadows. And, although I've gone a few rounds with parts of my shadow, I really hadn't touched upon its most hideous form. Until recently. But first, a little back-story.

Janice and I spent most of our time together. Not only did we share every morning and evening, but we also shared every working day. Being professors in the same department, our offices were only about fifty feet apart, and that meant that we talked from time to time each day, and even ate lunch together in one of our offices. That's a lot of togetherness, even for us.

That unusual closeness had its costs, and we both knew it. It was very hard, perhaps even impossible, to maintain separate identities with so much contact. And so we both, probably unconsciously, sacrificed some of who we were independent of each other for the joy of being together. I gave up being alone and, while that might not sound like any big deal, when you're as independent as I am, it *was* a big deal. I had become "lazy" academically, concentrating on what I was good at (intuitive ideas) and letting Janice do for me what I was not so good at (reviewing literature and making careful arguments). Most important, I had pushed aside my desire to become a better outlaw, mainly because outlaws, better and worse, had not worn well in Janice's psyche. Because being with Janice was such joy, I never thought much about it, but when I could no longer be with her I began recovering some of them. That felt good. Enter the shadow.

I sit in our living room, sipping a glass of cheap pink wine. I'm happy on this evening, and that's definitely a new feeling. So what's this all about? I begin to acknowledge how good it feels to be alone, to be academically productive, to practice being that better outlaw again. The last time I felt this free, I remember, was in Boulder in the mid-Seventies. At that time I was hoping Janice would join me there. But here, on this very ordinary evening, seven months after Janice died, I'm feeling optimistic about my future and excited about my present. I seem to have rediscovered a part of myself that I had misplaced.

Quite pleased with myself, I get up to let Mollie in, and then it hits. Unconsciously, did I want Janice to die? There it is—in all its horrific brutality—the darkest underbelly of my happiness. Now I know I did not give Janice cancer. I know, too, that I would not change one thing that I thought, felt, or did from the moment she was diagnosed until the second she died. What cuts so deeply is the possibility that I felt so constricted by Janice that I wished she would die so I could be free again to be myself. And then this line from Freud flashed before my eyes: "In almost every case where there is an intense emotional attachment to a particular person we find that behind the tender love there is a concealed hostility in the unconscious" (60). I sure as hell didn't need to remember that.

Until this morning, I told no one about this. Talking about your shadow is not the sort of thing you bring up over coffee. But this morning, Janice's best friend, Gale Young, called. It was her fifty-seventh birthday, and she called to thank me for a picture of Janice I'd sent her. After catching up, I eased into the hard stuff.

"With any luck, I should finish the last chapter of my book today."

"That's wonderful," Gale says. "Do you know how you're going to end it?"

"I think so. I don't know the order yet, but I'm going to talk about my shadow and then about moving my work into Janice's study. Both events will be tough to write and I really don't know which one to put first."

But Gale is much too intuitive to let this one slip by.

"Shadow? What shadow door are you going to open?"

And so I tell her. There's such a long silence that I think for a moment I've lost the connection. And then this.

"I really know that feeling. When I was married to Al, there were times that I wished he would die. That was the only way I could think of back then to get out of the marriage."

Another long pause.

"But then I told my analyst what I'd been feeling, and he said, 'There are probably parts of your relationship with Al that need to die, and I suspect he feels the same way. I think that's what your feeling is about. You contact it in its most undifferentiated form—wishing for the physical death of a loved one—but what the feeling really means is that some dysfunctional parts of your relationship should die. That's not a bad thing, really. That make sense?' Of course it did. Do you think that's what your feeling is all about? Do you think you wanted the more restrictive parts of your relationship with Janice to die? I would guess . . . no, I don't have to guess, I *know*, because we used to talk about it, that she wanted some aspects of her relationship with you to die."

I wipe a tear from my cheek, a tear that Gale cannot see, but can surely feel.

"Thanks, for more than you'll ever know. Maybe your shrink is giving us just a psychological rationalization for some ultimate evil in us, but until something better comes along, I'm buyin' it. And it feels right, as if I've begun, with your help, to sort out this shadow thing."

"Remember what Jung said," Gale reminds me. "If you can face your shadow, the really awful, terrible one, it can be the source of remarkable spiritual growth."

"He said that?"

"He did. And you'd better learn it if you intend to teach Janice's myth seminar," she adds, with a touch of lightness that we both need.

I cling to Gale's insight while still not letting go of my shadow. Some days it's easier to do than others.

As I continue to struggle with the varieties of grief, things are improving on the professional front. During Janice's final weeks, the faculty was wonderful. Some brought meals for ten and left them on our front porch. Others invited our out-of-town guests to stay in their homes. Still others car-pooled people around town, picked up groceries, and provided an endless supply of much-needed wine. After she died, our chair made a remarkable DVD retrospective of Janice's life for the memorial service. I began to see the faculty more as an extended family and less as a coven of adversaries. I finally realized how much they loved and respected Janice and the Board of Regents underscored this when they sent me a copy of their resolution celebrating Janice's scholarship, teaching, and community service.

Almost two years have passed between writing the last word of the previous paragraph and the first word of this one. I've spent most of that time keeping my last promise to Janice. Just before she slipped into a coma, I promised that I'd get her book published. After sending out sixty-seven proposals to literary agents all over the country, Sally van Haitsma of the Castiglia Literary Agency took on the project. After numerous revisions and updates, Mitch Allen of Left Coast Press, with warm support from Carolyn Ellis and Art Bochner, agreed to publish it. In record time, Mitch got it through production in time for the 2005 National Communication Association convention in Boston—a convention, I might add, at which Janice received posthumously the prestigious Douglas W. Ehninger Distinguished Rhetorical Scholar Award. Janice's book, *Erotic Mentoring: Women's Transformations in the University* is now a reality. I know she would be proud of it. I know I am. As Art Bochner said on the back cover: "Janice Rushing saved the best for last."

Performing Quality in Baby Steps

The life of the mind promises conversation; when it fails to deliver its disciples grow eccentric.

Vivian Gornick
Approaching Eye Level

Exactly three years ago today, Janice died. I have deliberately waited until today to begin this ending. I have moved into Janice's study and taken over her Macintosh G-4 (the "Big Mac"), which now sits in front of me. Behind me, not more than four feet away, is the couch where I spent those restless nights trying to stay alive. It is also the place where Janice spent her final days trying, but failing, to do the same thing. To my right, on a shelf between her myth books and her Jungian texts, I've created an informal shrine. It holds her picture, her book, her awards, a solid cedar heart a friend carved for her, a coffee cup from the family cabin saying "Love Is Kind," a gold necklace she bought in Dubrovnik, her wedding band and my mother's engagement ring, some sage we burned at her passing, and a heart-shaped jewelry box Gary Hawk made, now containing three remnants of her ashes—one for Mollie, one for me, and one for her. I feel her presence intensely in this place; it's almost too much sometimes, but then too, never quite enough.

As I write, a shaft of sun dances off my wedding band. It has been three years now, and any day someone is bound to ask how long I intend to wear it. I don't know what I'll say then, but I know what I'd say now. I'd say that my marriage to Janice did not end with her death. She may not be here physically, but her spirit infuses every corner of this sacred spot. She may have died, but our relationship has not. I read again one of the epigraphs in Art Bochner's tribute essay to Janice. It's by Robert Anderson and goes, "Death ends a life, but it does not end a relationship, which struggles on in the survivor's mind toward some final resolution, some clear meaning, which it perhaps never finds" ("Janice's Voice" 183). For now, I seek no final resolution, but as long as our connection is in my heart, the ring will stay on my finger.

Given all that's happened, it seems time to reflect a bit on what I've tried to do. I began writing seven years ago, in 2000, after being diagnosed with cancer. Like any traumatic experience, cancer threw my life into chaos. This story is my attempt to make sense of my life and to provide narrative continuity for what may be left of it. Because I wanted what is ahead to be better than what was behind, I modeled my own journey as a quest for Quality, much like Robert M. Pirsig did in *Zen and the Art of Motorcycle Maintenance*. I could find Quality most easily, *Zen* taught me, by caring passionately about what I do, because that sort of intense commitment erases, if only for a moment, the rational split between me-as-subject and other-as-object. But whereas Pirsig's alter ego, Phaedrus, attacked the rational structures in the academy with the savagery of a wolf, I struggled to transform my own wolfish nature as a professor (a low quality animal in the university) into a coyote, the trickster of mythology (a higher quality creature in the academy).

I learned the trade of a trickster early in life from my Aunt Hilda and, to some extent, in reaction to my father's own wolfishness. But somewhere along the way, I lost the trickster and vacillated between dependent sheep and my father's raging wolf. I began to rediscover my trickster, somewhat ironically, within an even more rigid social hierarchy than the academy—namely, the medical profession that dealt with my cancer. By inviting them to join me in imagination, where their superior medical knowledge was offset by my outrageous tricksterness, I was able to receive the treatment I needed while never compromising the humanity I valued—high quality experiences. But it was one thing to be the coyote/trickster with medical practitioners meeting me for the first time and quite another to act that way with academic colleagues who had known me for all too long as the wolf. My struggle, then as now, was to transform myself from the wolf that seeks to destroy academic structures to the coyote that seeks to destabilize them. As the end of my tale implies, I still have good days and bad, for wolves die hard and coyotes emerge slowly from the womb.

So that's my story in bold strokes. Now for a few nuances. On one level, I am writing to find my voice, the sound of me on the page. Back there in Chapter 6, I groused a lot about not having a voice, or, better put, having the homogenized, depersonalized voice of the traditional scholar constricted by the rules and conventions of academic writing. I sound better now. As I re-read these pages, I smile because I sound more like I envision myself even when I'm not writing. And I thank all of the ethnographers who, in different ways and to differing degrees, promised me that when my feelings and intuitions joined up with my thoughts, I'd like the outcome. They were right.

Now I want to expand the scope of my voice. I'll continue writing autoethnographies, in fact I've already begun a few, but unlike many who make "the ethnographic turn" and never turn back, I intend to turn back. Not completely, of course. I'll never do "measure it and treasure it" social science again, but I do want to carry my enhanced sound system forward into interpretive work in rhetoric and film studies. Maybe I'm still trying to satisfy that cranky critic who once said that whereas I had no voice, those with whom I wrote did. But I think it's more than that. Although I didn't realize it at the time, my "mini-critique" of Guy Clark's "The Randall Knife" fused two forms of scholarship (rhetorical criticism and autoethnography) that are usually light years apart. Here is at least one way to transcend some of those traditional oppositions in academic life.

But what about those other oppositions, the more personal ones? As Art Bochner, my most insightful and compassionate critic, constantly reminds me, the narrative energy of my tale all but feeds on preserving and even creating—not transcending or unraveling—oppositions. It is me against the chairpersons, me against the administrators, me against the letter writers, me against the writing conventions, me against co-authors, me against medical practitioners, hell, even me against some students. For someone who promised from the outset that autoethnographic writing would collapse such oppositions, there's more than a little hypocrisy creeping in here. Perhaps some finer discriminations need to be made. I think to contest the dehumanization brought on by organizational hierarchy, some opposition is necessary, but it can, and should, be a *relational* opposition, not an individual opposition. As

I've demonstrated time and time again, wolves use rage to destroy others for their shortcomings (individual opposition), while coyotes use humor to help others soften their shortcomings (relational opposition). These days I'm into modifying shortcomings.

Here's a recent example. Our department had a new tenure-track position and, with a little trickster magic, I conned my way into being appointed search committee chair. I saw this as an opportunity to show my colleagues that I could do more than just snarl about their shortcomings. And so I kicked my latent OCD into overdrive, received and responded to each of almost forty applicants instantly, and organized things such that everyone could keep pace with what was going on. I remember whispering to our first choice, during her on-campus interview, that if she were offered the job and accepted, I'd buy her a bottle of over-priced scotch and marry her mother for a least a year, then we'd re-evaluate. This trickster act, violating almost every sanction of structural rationality, worked like a charm. She took the position. I don't want to make too much of this, or get too inflated over my newfound collegiality, but I think my trickster efforts on the department's behalf were both noticed and appreciated. Not an earth-shaking change, to be sure, but, as the line goes in the film *What About Bob?*, "baby steps," the only way to begin. A little less wolf, a little more coyote.

My thoughts on the academy are at the baby-steps level too, but those steps are more complicated. Earlier I spoke of the Church of Reason, Pirsig's metaphor for the university in *Zen*. Exploring that metaphor in more detail serves as a prelude to my evolving sense of university life.

In describing the sort of rationality his alter ego Phaedrus worked within and later attacked in the name of Quality, Pirsig writes:

> His kind of rationality has been used since antiquity to remove
> oneself from the tedium and depression of one's immediate sur-
> roundings. What makes it hard to see is that where once it was
> used to get away from it all, the escape has been so successful
> that now it is the "it all" that the romantics are trying to escape.
> What makes his world so hard to see clearly is not its strange-
> ness but its usualness. Familiarity can blind you too. (63)

Although Pirsig doesn't elaborate, the "tedium and depression of one's immediate surroundings" means all the rest of the messy business of living—relationships, feelings, spiritual longings, bodily desires, and the like. Pirsig is right when he notes that, since classical antiquity, rationality and its technological offshoots have been privileged by intellectuals over those "lesser qualities" that dominate the great unwashed.

Not much has changed over the years. A colleague still greets new graduate students with the rather lyrical line, "Welcome to the life of the mind." On the surface, an innocent enough aphorism, but underneath a subtle reaffirmation that university life is only about the head, about developing just the rational potentials of students. This myopic commitment to the reasoning mind (as opposed, for example, to the sentient body), is the most longstanding, most deeply entrenched, and most intractable legacy of reason within the academy. Anyone who dares question this foundational belief, and who might open the academy to more holistic, embodied, or emotional ways of learning and knowing, is derided and, whenever possible, excommunicated by Church officials. "The strength of the taboo," writes Jane Tompkins, who has experienced more than her fair share of such derision, "can be gauged by the academician's inevitable recourse to name-calling when emotion, spirituality, and imagination are brought into the curricular conversation: 'touchy-feely,' 'soft,' 'unrigorous,' 'mystical,' 'therapeutic,' and 'Mickey Mouse' are the all-time favorites, with 'psychobabble' and 'bullshit' being not far behind" (214).

So what exactly is this "it all" of rationality that, like the invisibility of smog when you're in it, erodes the quality of university life and yet is so fiercely guarded by Church officialdom? In a phrase, it is analytical thinking, reducing the totality of life to a series of either/ors, subjects or objects, ones or zeroes, offs or ons. For Pirsig, this either/or reality seems so natural that we come to believe it represents the true nature of things. This very dialectical process is what Plato used long ago to destroy Quality and the sophists who taught rhetoric. In many ways the continuing division of cultures into ever more minute parts has given us the fragmentation known as the postmodern condition. The most basic of these divisions and the one most difficult to see, is the cleavage between immediate surface appearance and reflective underlying form, an unseen separation that produces two incommensurable forms of reality, classical and romantic (Pirsig 60–61). As Pirsig notes, the cultural impact of this division has been devastating:

At present we're snowed under with an irrational expansion of blind data-gathering in the sciences because there's no rational format for any understanding of scientific creativity. At present we are also snowed under with a lot of stylishness in the arts—thin art—because there's very little assimilation or extension into underlying form. We have artists with no scientific knowledge, scientists with no artistic knowledge, and both with no spiritual sense of gravity at all, and the result is not just bad, it is ghastly. (264)

Although these oppositions are so ubiquitous that they define "meaningfulness" in language, they were born in the academies of classic antiquity, those schools that gave us Western Civilization. Is it any wonder that reason is so hard to challenge or change within the academy? And so "it all" emerges as the rationally constructed oppositions and their attendant hierarchies that define the structure of contemporary life. This is the life of the mind, and because the mind is the only thing left living, the rest of the person (body, feelings, soul) often dies—a very low quality trade off.

But turnabout is (un)fair play, and what the university once gave to culture writ large, culture has now given back in spades. For if "reason gone wild" has produced cultures whose meanings and values are locked into its hierarchical structures, themselves generated by rational divisions, those very structures, always present within the university to some degree, have now come to dominate it. Tompkins again captures the specificity of the problem in academia:

Throughout this discussion of the compartmentalization of learning, two themes have been running parallel to each other. One concerns the intense focus on performance, geared to the perceived necessity of gaining a foothold in a fiercely competitive marketplace; the other concerns higher education's exclusive emphasis on intellectual development. As things stand now, these two emphases reinforce one another; there are very few ways to excel academically, and thus to become marketable, that include attention to creativity, self-knowledge, and compassion for oneself and others. (214)

Put another way, universities have become indistinguishable from corporations; the corporate structures of the medical profession have gotten a lot of press in my story. This turnabout has not exactly been positive for many who work within universities. John Rodden, who I have mentioned earlier in several contexts, sounded a warning way back in 1993:

> At our "Research I" institutions, the transformation from ivory
> tower to industrial park is almost complete. The gentleman [sic]
> scholar and absent-minded professor have given way to the
> knowledge technician and the academic entrepreneur. Even in
> its failed aspirations, the multiuniversity no longer wishes to
> become an organic society of intellectuals. It is simply an aca-
> demic-industrial complex conducting a variety of profit-making
> activities like any other large corporation. We are losing all belief
> that living the intellectual life in the academy is not just a career
> but a *calling*. (126)

To underscore the sinister pervasiveness of the classical/romantic split, both Tompkins and Rodden's poignant critiques presuppose it. It's not hard to see how the very language used to craft their complaints reproduces the underlying forms of classical understanding, while their wistful longing for a university comprised of an organic society of intellectuals who might be there from some "calling" are vestiges of the surface immediacy of romantic understanding.

So what, if anything, can be done to change, or at least challenge, this massive philosophical split that creates the university's myopic commitment to reason and its gradual conversion from an academy to a corporation? I'm not sure, really, but my trickster has been playing around with three rhetorical strategies that have shown some signs of success.

The first grows out of Kenneth Burke's comments on mystery in hierarchy, admittedly a grandiose way to begin.

> [W]e might begin with the proposition that mystery arises at
> that point where different *kinds* of beings are in communication.
> In mystery there must be *strangeness*; but the estranged must
> also be thought of as in some way capable of communion. . . .
> [T]he conditions for "mystery" are set by *any* pronounced social
> distinctions, as between nobility and commoners, courtiers and
> king, leader and people, rich and poor, judge and prisoner at the
> bar, "superior race" and underprivileged "races" or minorities.
> (*Rhetoric* 115)

It's not hard to pinpoint the sources of mystery in my tale. Physicians and university professors are typically called "doctor," while their patients and students, respectively, are called something else, something less. But if Burke is right, there must be, even in this status difference, some means toward communion, toward lessening the gap between those who have/know more and those who have/know less. For me, communion can at least be approached through name changes.

Recall that I always called my mother and father by their first names, Jo and Ted rather than Mom and Dad. Even as a young trickster-in-training, I seemed to intuit that calling my parents by their proper names rather than their culturally proscribed titles would lessen the mystery between us. I've done that with all doctors throughout my story. I've always called both medical doctors and my academic colleagues by their first names rather than by their status titles. In many ways, I use this strategy as a litmus test. Over the years, I've found that those who get all uptight with the first name thing are usually those who are not secure enough in who they are or with what they do to relate to me as a person rather than as a position. By contrast, those who welcome and even initiate (and many do) this gentle deflating of difference are those I've learned I can trust. Now, some departments in which I've worked operate on a first-name basis simply as a matter of course, but some don't. And those that don't need a trickster more than those that do.

Because tricksters are teachers, I try to instill this strategy in my students as well. But that's not always easy. When speaking of my colleagues, I always refer to them by their first names, never as Dr. This or Dr. That. Most students are reasonably comfortable with this. It is when I get personal that some sphincter muscles begin to tighten. When I was younger, I used to insist that students call me Tom rather than Dr. Frentz. But I was naïve about the strength of cultural conditioning in some parts of the country. I didn't realize how deeply engrained respect virtually mandated addressing others by their formal titles. So now I say "You can call me anything you're comfortable with except perhaps 'Shitface.' That term of endearment comes from my father." When I'm really feeling playful, I go for the compromise, "How does Dr. Tom sound to you?" That one has had, I must admit, mixed results. As yet, no one has suggested Dr. Shitface, but I suppose if somebody ever does, I'll have to consider it.

A second strategy I use to demystify academic hierarchies was born in *Zen*. In the 1950s, Pirsig's Phaedrus felt nothing but contempt for the well-scrubbed, bright-eyed grade grubbers in the front rows of his classes, while he identified completely with the angry, unkempt, wolf-like radicals who sat in the back and always failed. He worried about this once to his artist friend, Robert DeWeese. "Well, there's something whacky here . . . because the students I like the most, the ones I really feel a sense of identity with, are all *failing!*" (123). At the time, DeWeese just roared with laughter, but later Phaedrus came to see that what he'd said was a kind of supertruth. "The best students always *are* flunking. *Every* good teacher knows that," he mused (124). They are failing, of course, because they refuse to be sheep and play by the rules of reason, and every good teacher, Phaedrus implies, empathizes with the courage of those would-be wolves who refuse to get an education at the cost of their humanity.

But, although Phaedrus may have identified with his failing students, he still failed them. I don't fail them, I recruit them—not to be grownup wolves, no future there, but to be tricksters, to learn the rules, figure out how to slide around the most dehumanizing of them, and still get an education with their humanity intact. Here's how I work it. The trickster says: "The more information *about* the system is shared with people *in* the system, the less that information can be used to dominate the people in the system." This is because information that faculty has but students don't have can be used in ways that are not always in the best interests of the students. If students have that information, the hierarchy is preserved but destabilized, and the students acquire more flexibility in determining their own academic destinies. As hierarchy softens, the mystery embodied in it lessens. And so, from time to time, with students who show a little trickster aptitude, I share information about how the department works. Nothing sinister, nothing personal, no backstage gossip, just some of the more discretionary policies that are not printed in the *Manual of Graduate Studies*. I'm sure that some of my colleagues would prefer that I didn't do this, but I look on these trickster acts as arming students with "equipment for living," as Kenneth Burke once said ("Literature" 304). And for me, that's high quality equipment.

By far the most effective strategy to destabilize hierarchy and reduce mystery surrounds the autoethnography seminar I now teach. You don't even have to be a trickster to do this one. Before I elaborate on my approach to autoethnography, three qualifications are in order. First, I am certainly not claiming that autoethnographic approaches to education are a radical way to replace 2,500 years of Western Civilization's love affair with reason. Second, I am not maintaining that autoethnographic methods are the only, or even the most effective, way to recontextualize rationality within the academy. Before devolving, Pirsig's Phaedrus stumbled upon numerous creative methods for teaching Quality in his rhetoric (English composition) classes (184–96). Jane Tompkins' own innovative teaching strategies offer another set of alternatives, while Laurel Richardson's creative approaches to sociological writing provide still another (Richardson). Finally, I am not saying that my own personal version of these methods is the way everyone should proceed. Again, Art Bochner, Carolyn Ellis, Bud Goodall, Ron Pelias, and a host of others in communication, anthropology, and sociology offer productive variations on the autoethnographic theme (Bochner and Ellis; Ellis *Ethnographic I*; Ellis and Bochner; Goodall; Pelias). But I am claiming that autoethnographic writing and the thinking/feeling that accompanies it can fuse students' inner and outer selves—their hearts with their minds—and that such fusions can be a very high quality form of learning and doing. I didn't see this initially, but stumbled upon it over time as the course evolved and I began to see what worked and what didn't. Here's how it all came about.

Like Alasdair MacIntyre and many others, I assume that life only becomes fully meaningful when it is experienced as an ongoing narrative. Life does not happen as a story, not even the life of the mind, but rather must be crafted into one by those who live it. Again, echoing a long tradition in numerous academic disciplines and other walks of life, I've tried to do that here by combining the isolated incidents of my cancer and academic experiences into a narrative whole, one that I hope leads somewhere productive for me, the storyteller, and for you, the reader. But, although most of us experience our lives as ongoing stories, our tales, like this one, do not evolve seamlessly without disruptions and intrusions. Occasionally, a life event—like going insane for Pirsig's Phaedrus, or like my being diagnosed with cancer, then losing Janice to cancer—tears the narrative thread of our lives, and, when it does, there is always an opportunity either for productive growth or destructive regression.

It is that opportunity that I've tried to exploit in the lives of my ethnography students. "If you can go back to that time when something tossed your life into turmoil and feel now what you felt back then, perhaps you can re-story that event from where you are now, not to 'make it go away,' but rather to change what it means in your larger life story," I tell them. This is an inward challenge, a move toward the heart, that invites students to do what they are rarely invited to do in the university—to see their personal lives as an integral part of their educational experience. For many, it is a foreboding challenge. Not all 23-year-olds, I have discovered, have experienced life-altering events, and even those who have often find it easier to suppress the experiences rather than to relive them in writing. Sometimes students work with things as ordinary as the breakup of a high school romance, but I've learned there is no universal standard for what counts as a life-altering event. For many students, an early romantic failure feels just as traumatic as going mad or discovering they have cancer. The nature of the event is not as important as mustering the courage and the skill to revisit it emotionally and subjectively. This is one small interior step in recovering from the academy's addiction to rationality.

A second step is to encourage students to find, contact, and talk with other characters in their story, the very people who were involved with the original traumatic experience. This is an outer move, but still grounded in feelings. For me, it was chatting with medical professionals and academic colleagues to hear the mistrust they harbored, feel the fears they felt, and experience the anger they reflected back to me. For many students, it involves contacting ex-lovers or spouses, abusive parents, neglected grandparents, surviving family members, domineering clergy, even former inmates, the list is endless. Many contacts fail because others are unwilling and/or unable to revisit the experience the students are dealing with. Others fail because contact does little more than reactivate the destructive relationship patterns that produced the original trauma. But some succeed, in part because, like the ethnographic student, the relevant others are also not where they were psychologically when the event in question occurred. When this occurs, students use classroom experiences to improve some aspects of their lives outside the classroom. Here's one small way to honor Art Bochner's plea to reintegrate the personal and professional lives within the university ("Divided") and to open social science to multiple perspectives on cultural life ("Narratives"), both clearly high quality aspirations.

Students ultimately re-story their lives by rewriting an event that once disrupted them, much as I have tried to do here. This seminar is, to be sure, only one small way to move beyond the classical/romantic split in an institution so committed to reproduce it. But if enough of us begin taking those first steps, perhaps more will learn how to walk on their own—not rejecting reason, but with more than just reason and with a larger understanding of what reason can be. I keep thinking that autoethnographic writing, much like fiction writing, might begin to heal the enormous rift between classical and romantic understanding that so bedeviled Pirsig's Phaedrus. When these writings work, the stories students tell change the evolving surface of their lives by rethinking their underlying form. As one example among many, a young woman in my class, after reflecting on a long-term abusive relationship and mustering the courage to talk with the perpetrator, recognized that she had connected physical violence to sexual arousal for years. Writing her way into this truth was a first step to breaking that dysfunctional connection in her relational life.

These are only three of the trickster steps that I've taken so far. How many more are still to come? Although I still use trickster tricks to delight students, these days my goal is much more serious. I suppose, if I'm completely honest here, there's a bit of the shepherd creeping in here, but with an important difference. Most shepherds try to reproduce hierarchy: I try to renew it.

I've risked "talking academic" as I conclude this because I care deeply about changing some of the more dehumanizing things about the academy, and to even *think* about doing that entails talking the talk. for just a bit. I want to end with some of my own talk. It is something mythic that Janice and I said years ago that feels right to say again here. We had been speaking of two Greek gods—Apollo, the heavenly god of light and reason, and his more earthly twin, the dark and sensuous Dionysus—arguing that worshipping Apollo and repressing Dionysus leads to a low quality of life in the academy. And then from a source Pirsig would surely appreciate, we shared these thoughts:

> In the allegory of the horses and chariot in Plato's *Phaedrus*, the person is the charioteer, the planning, calculating *logistikon* who cannot go where he wants to go without the non-intellectual elements of emotion and appetite. These wilder passions guide him toward understanding by being responsive to such things as beauty and deep feeling. They provide insight as to where goodness is, and the motivating drive to move the soul to find it. . . .
> If it is our compulsion towards speed and height that renders us immobile and hinders our vision, then it is only by propitiating the shunned dark god and not by stepping up that we will see where we want to go. (244)

I see these words now, though I did not when I helped write them, as still another call to Quality. I think it's time to story up a little resurrection. I've tried to write part of my own revival here; you'll have to write your own somewhere else. I hope Dionysus more than Apollo is your guide. "What is best?"

Zen's narrator asked to guide his story. Even now, I'm not sure I know. But I do know that, for both of us, "what is best" entailed suffering through "what is worst." Pirsig lost Chris; I lost Janice. Perhaps we all must fall down before we can get up.

This being the third of my three "last chapters," I think it's time—perhaps way past time—to wrap things up. But how? When faced with a similar dilemma, Richard Quinney once wrote, "To be true to the [ethnographic] genre is to realize that the ethnography ends only with the death of the ethnographer. We write, in the meantime, to save our lives" (380). Words no cancer survivor wants to hear. I hope there is not some macabre irony at work here. For, even as I finish, I face hip replacement surgery in two weeks. My surgeon wrote on his diagnosis, "Advanced osteoarthritis of the left hip with a fairly large cyst formation at the superior acetabulum." The hip deal I get, but what's this about a large cyst? Now the surgeon assures me that "cyst" is just a medical term for some arthritic deterioration of bone matter in my hip, not a synonym for "tumor," and that he'll remove it during the procedure. But since this cyst is right across from where my cancerous lymph nodes once were, there's still some anxiety. I don't want to end my ethnography by fulfilling Richard Quinney's prophesy. But I don't think that will happen. After sharing my fears with Jane Sutton in correspondence, a dear friend and wild feminist rhetorician, Jane, who talks with angels, wrote back with a passion and conviction that I couldn't ignore: "It's not your time, Tom."

More words to live by, I hope.

Works Cited

Anderson, Robert. *I Never Sang for my Father: A Play in Two Acts*. New York: Dramatists Play Series, Inc., 1968.

Blade Runner. Dir. Ridley Scott. The Ladd Company/Sir Run Run Shaw, 1982.

Bly, Robert. *Iron John: A Book about Men*. Reading, MA: Addison-Wesley, 1990.

Bochner, Arthur P. "It's About Time: Narrative and the Divided Self." *Qualitative Inquiry* 3 (1997): 418–438.

_____. "Narratives Virtues." *Qualitative Inquiry* 7 (2001): 131–157.

_____. "Janice's Voice." *Southern Communication Journal* 71 (June 2006): 183–193.

Burke, Kenneth, *A Rhetoric of Motives*. Berkeley, CA: University of California Press, 1969.

_____. "Dramatism." *International Encyclopedia of Social Sciences*. Ed. David L. Sills. New York: Macmillan/Free Press, 1968. 445–452.

_____. "Literature as Equipment for Living." *The Philosophy of Literary Form*. Berkeley: University of California Press, 1973. 293–304.

Butch Cassidy and the Sundance Kid. Dir. George Roy Hill. Fox, 1969.

Campbell, Joseph. *The Hero with a Thousand Faces*. New York: Bollingen Series/Princeton University Press, 1972.

Clark, Guy. "Anyhow, I Love You." Perf. Guy Clark with Emmylou Harris, Rodney Crowell, and Waylon Jennings. *Texas Cookin'*. RCA Studios, 1976.

_____. "Crystelle." Perf. Guy Clark. *The South Coast of Texas*. Warner Bros. Records, Inc., 1981.

_____. "The Randall Knife." Perf. Guy Clark. *Better Days*. Warner Bros. Records, Inc., 1983.

Composing Ethnography: Alternative Forms of Qualitative Writing. Eds. Carolyn Ellis and Arthur P. Bochner. Walnut Creek, CA: AltaMira Press, 1996.

Crawford, Lyle. "Personal Ethnography." *Communication Monographs* 63 (1996): 158–170.

Eco, Umberto. *The Name of the Rose.* Trans. William Weaver. New York: Bantam Books, 1984.

Ellis, Carolyn and Arthur P. Bochner. "Autoethnography, Personal Narrative, Reflexivity: Researcher as Subject." *Handbook of Qualitative Research.* Eds. Norman Denzin and Yvonna Lincoln. Beverly Hills, CA: Sage Publications, 2000. 733–768.

Ellis, Carolyn. "'There are Survivors': Telling a Story of Sudden Death." *Sociological Quarterly* 34 (1993): 711–730.

_____. "Sociological Introspection and Emotional Experience." *Symbolic Interaction* 14 (1991): 23–50.

_____. *The Ethnographic I: A Methodological Novel About Autoethnography.* Walnut Creek, CA: AltaMira Press, 2004.

Emerson, Richard M. "Power-Dependence Relations." *American Sociological Review* 27 (1962): 31–41.

Ethnographically Speaking: Autoethnography, Literature, and Aesthetics. Eds. Arthur P. Bochner and Carolyn Ellis. Walnut Creek, CA: AltaMira Press, 2002.

Farrell, Thomas B. and Thomas S. Frentz. "Communication and Meaning: A Language-Action Synthesis." *Philosophy and Rhetoric* 12 (1979): 215–255.

Farrell, Thomas B. "Aspects of Coherence in Conversation and Rhetoric." *Conversational Coherence: Form, Structure, and Strategy.* Eds. Robert T. Craig and Karen Tracy. Beverly Hills, CA: Sage Publications, 1983. 259–284.

Frank, Arthur W. *At the Will of the Body: Reflections on Illness.* New York: Houghton Mifflin Company, 1991.

Frentz, Thomas. "Ashes of Love." *Southern Communication Journal* 71 (Summer 2006): 195–203.

Frentz, Thomas S. "Resurrecting the Feminine in *The Name of the Rose*." *PRE/TEXT* 9 (1988): 123–145.

_____. "Rhetoric and Public Address Division Minutes of April 6, 2002." *C-O-N-N-E-C-T-I-O-N-S* 22 (Summer, 2002): 35.

_____. "Rhetoric and Public Address Division Minutes: Uncut, Uncensored, and Undeniable." *C-O-N-N-E-C-T-I-O-N-S* 20 (Summer, 2001): 28–29.

_____. "Rhetorical Conversation, Time, and Moral Action." *Quarterly Journal of Speech* 71 (1985): 1–18.

_____. "The Unbearable Darkness of Seeing." *C-O-N-N-E-C-T-I-O-N-S* 14 (1985): 1, 11, 19.

Frentz, Tom. "Three Tributes to Janice." Unpublished memorial service remarks, March 26, 2004.

Freud, Sigmund. *Totem and Taboo*. Trans. James Strachey. New York: W. W. Norton & Company, 1913/1950.

Goodall, H. Lloyd, Jr. *Writing the New Ethnography*. Lanham, Maryland: AltaMira Press, 2000.

Gornick, Vivian. *Approaching Eye Level*. Boston: Beacon Press, 1996.

Hyde, Lewis. *Trickster Makes This World: Mischief, Myth, and Art*. New York: Farrar, Straus and Giroux, 1998.

Jung, C. G. *Four Archetypes: Mother, Rebirth, Spirit, Trickster*. Trans. R. F. C. Hull. Bollingen Ser. XX. Princeton: Princeton UP, 1959/1969.

_____. *Memories, Dreams, Reflections*. Trans. Richard and Clara Winston. New York: Vintage Books, 1965.

_____. *The Portable Jung*. Ed. Joseph Campbell. Trans. R. F. C. Hull. New York: Viking, 1971.

Lamott, Anne. *Bird by Bird: Some Instructions on Writing and Life*. New York: Anchor Books, 1995.

Le Guin, Ursula K. *A Wizard of Earthsea*. New York: Bantam Books, 1975.

Leonard, Scott, and Michael McClure. *Myth & Knowing: An Introduction to World Mythology*. New York: McGraw-Hill, 2004.

MacIntyre, Alasdair. *After Virtue: A Study in Moral Theory*. Notre Dame, IN: University of Notre Dame Press, 1981.

Neumann, Erich. *The Great Mother: An Analysis of the Archetype*. Trans. Ralph Manheim. Bollingen Ser. XLVII. Princeton: Princeton University Press, 1972.

Nussbaum, Martha C. *The Fragility of Goodness: Luck and Ethics in Greek Tragedy and Philosophy*. Cambridge: Cambridge University Press, 1986.

Pelias, Ronald J. *Writing Performance: Poeticizing the Researcher's Body*. Carbondale: Southern Illinois University Press, 1999.

Pirsig, Robert M. *Zen and the Art of Motorcycle Maintenance: An Inquiry into Values*. New York: Bantam Books, 1975.

Plato. *Phaedrus*. Trans. W. C. Helmbold and W. G. Rabinowitz. New York: The Bobbs-Merrill Company, Inc., 1956.

Quinney, Richard. "Once My Father Traveled West to California." *Composing Ethnography: Alternative Forms of Qualitative Writing*. Eds. Carolyn Ellis and Arthur P. Bochner. Walnut Creek, CA: AltaMira Press, 1996. 357–382.

Radin, Paul. *The Trickster: A Study in American Indian Mythology*. New York: Bell Publishing Company, Inc., 1956.

Rodden, John. "Field of Dreams." *Western Journal of Communication* 57 (1993): 111–138.

Rose. Dan. *Living the Ethnographic Life*. Thousand Oaks, CA: Sage, 1990.

Richardson, Laurel. *Fields of Play: Constructing an Academic Life*. New Brunswick, NJ: Rutgers University Press, 1997.

Rushing, Janice Hocker, and Thomas S. Frentz. "The Gods Must Be Crazy: The Denial of Descent in Academic Scholarship." *Quarterly Journal of Speech* 85 (1999): 229–246.

Rushing, Janice Hocker. *Erotic Mentoring: Women's Transformations in the University*. Walnut Creek, CA: Left Coast Press, 2006.

_____. "Evolution of 'The New Frontier' in *Alien* and *Aliens*: Patriarchal Co-optation of the Feminine Archetype." *Quarterly Journal of Speech* 75 (1989): 1–24.

Sabo, Deborah. "For Janice." Unpublished poem, February 20, 2004.

Shelly, Mary. *Frankenstein*. New York: Bantam Books, 1818/1991.

Tompkins, Jane. *A Life in School: What the Teacher Learned*. Reading, MA: Addison-Wesley, 1996.

Turner, Victor. *From Ritual to Theatre: The Human Seriousness of Play*. New York: Performing Arts Journal Publications, 1982.

Index

Rushing, Janice Hocker, 52, 57–60, 65–66, 73–78,159–172, 182
cancer, 159–163
Douglas W. Ehninger Distinguished Rhetorical Scholar Award, 170
memorial service, 164–167

Sabo, Deborah, 159
shape-shifter, 23, 61
sheep, 21, 28–29, 39, 45, 49, 76–77, 86, 102, 105, 109, 179
sheep speak, 51–60, 107, 124
Shelby, Carroll, 32
Shelly, Mary, 101
shepherd, 21, 45, 47, 54–55, 58–60, 63, 67, 71, 86, 102, 106–109, 113, 115, 119, 182
"Sociological Introspection and Emotional Experience"(Ellis), 27
Socrates, 49
Southern Communication Journal,166
Starhawk, 114
structure, 22
departmental, 117, 136
Stuckey, Mary, 151
Sutton, Jane, 183

TA's, 118–121
Ted (father), 27, 31–37, 41–42, 45, 54, 157–158, 178
cancer, 41
Terhune, Albert Peyson, 29
"'There are Survivors': Telling a Story of Sudden Death" (Ellis), 18
Three Tributes to Janice" (Frentz), 164
Tompkins, Jane, 103, 175–176, 180
Totem and Taboo (Freud), 168
trickster, 22–23, 28, 34, 39, 45, 61, 78, 88, 91–93, 98, 103, 105–106, 109, 119, 121, 124, 174, 179
coyote, 61, 172
Loki, 61
three steps to, 180–182

The Trickster: A Study in American Indian Mythology (Radin), 23
Trickster Makes This World: Mischief, Myth, and Art (Hyde), 22, 43, 104
Turner, Victor, 22–23, 119

"The Unbearable Darkness of Seeing" (Frentz), 107
The Unbearable Lightness of Being (Kundera), 107

voice, personal ethnographic, 150, 173
von Haitsma, Sally, 170

Whitebear, Tom, 158
Williams, Fred, 45–48, 51–52, 109–111, 114
Wilmot, Bill, 133–135, 153
Wily E. Coyote, 22, 43
A Wizard of Earthsea (Le Guin), 107
wolf, 21–22,28,37,45,47,51–52, 61, 77, 82,102,105, 109, 119, 124, 136, 148, 174
as Phaedrus, 62, 172
canis latrans, 22
canus lupus, 43
radicals, 179
relate as, 76
Woodward, Malcolm, 162
Writing the New Ethnography (Goodall), 23

Young, Gale, 161–162, 168–169

Zen and the Art of Motorcycle Maintenance: An Inquiry into Values (Pirsig), 13, 20–22, 39, 61–63, 117, 144, 158, 172, 175, 178–180, 183

About the Author

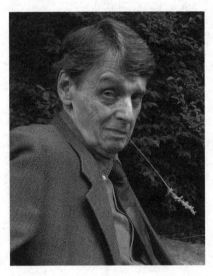

Thomas S. Frentz is a professor of Communication at the University of Arkansas, Fayetteville. An eclectic scholar in both the social sciences and humanities, he has published three books, twenty-nine scholarly articles, four book chapters, over fifty convention papers, and has lectured extensively at colleges and universities across the country. He teaches courses in rhetorical theory, criticism, film, ethnography, and myth. In 1994/1995 he served as president of the Southern States Communication Association. In 2006 he was named Master Researcher by the J. William Fulbright College of Arts and Sciences at the University of Arkansas. In 2007 the Rhetoric and Communication Theory division of the National Communication Association named him Distinguished Scholar of 2007. He lives in Fayetteville with his cat, Mollie.